Come Hungry

Cookbook

Explore The Home Cook 41 Simple Recipes to Know by Heart

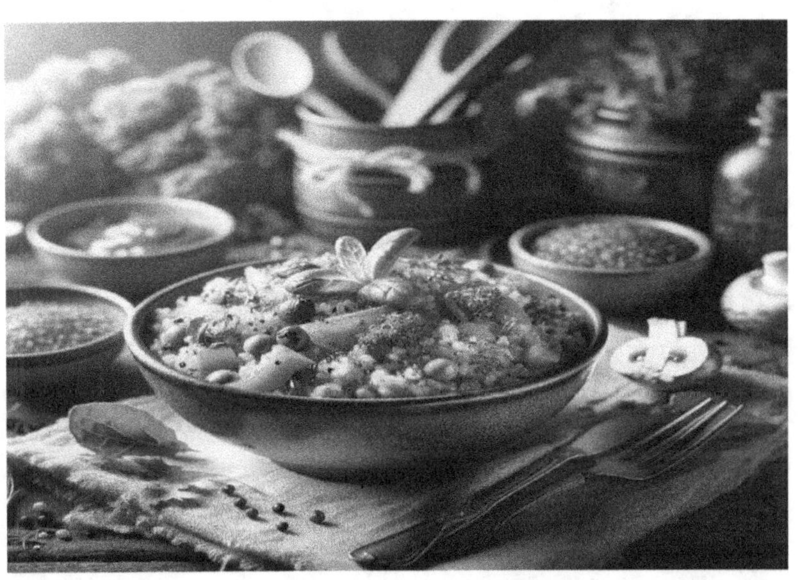

Benedict Robinson

TABLE OF CONTENTS

How to Use This Cookbook

Explore and Choose a Recipe: Start by browsing through the cookbook to explore the different recipes it offers. Each recipe will likely introduce you to flavors from various parts of the world. Choose one that appeals to your taste preferences or intrigues you.

Read the Recipe Thoroughly: Before you start cooking, read the entire recipe from start to finish. This will give you a clear understanding of the ingredients you need, the equipment required, and the steps involved. Pay attention to serving sizes, preparation times, and any special techniques mentioned.

Gather Ingredients and Equipment: Collect all the ingredients listed in the recipe. It is best to use fresh ingredients for the best flavor. Also, ensure you have all the necessary kitchen equipment and tools on hand, such as pots, pans, knives, and measuring cups/spoons.

Follow the Recipe Steps: Proceed by following the recipe step-by-step. Pay attention to details like cooking times, temperatures, and sequence of adding ingredients. These cookbooks are usually designed to be user-friendly, so the steps should be easy to follow.

Serve and Enjoy: Once you have finished cooking, serve the dish according to the recipe's suggestions.

Many recipes also include tips for garnishing or serving suggestions to enhance the dish's presentation and taste.

Bonus Tips:
If you are unfamiliar with any techniques or terms used in the recipe, don't hesitate to look them up for clarification or send us an email - healthyreadspublisher@gmail.com

Feel free to make slight modifications to suit your dietary needs or flavor preferences.
Enjoy the process of cooking and the journey of tasting new flavors!

Remember, cookbooks like this are not only about following recipes but also about exploring and enjoying a variety of cultures and cuisines. Happy cooking!

INTRODUCTION

Embracing the Joys of Simple, Flavorful Cooking

The Come Hungry Cookbook: This is not simply a list of recipes; rather, it is an invitation to embark on a delightful and gastronomic adventure, appropriate for cooks of all skill levels who want simplicity without compromising flavor.

It can be difficult to find time to cook in today's hectic world, but there is nothing quite like preparing and enjoying a home-cooked meal. This cookbook, which includes 41 simple dishes that will hopefully bring delicious flavors to your table with little effort, is your travel companion.

Each recipe in this book has been carefully curated not just for its simplicity and taste, but also for the experience it offers. Whether you are a seasoned cook or just starting out, these dishes will inspire you to explore new flavors while appreciating the beauty of simple, wholesome ingredients.

From tantalizing toasts and fresh salads to hearty grain dishes and quick dinners, every recipe is designed to maximize flavor while minimizing time spent in the kitchen. The homemade dressings and artisan breads will add a special touch to your meals, turning everyday cooking into a delightful experience.

This book also celebrates the variety of cooks in the kitchen. The recipes offer a flavor of different cultures and traditions, drawing inspiration from a wide range of cuisines. It is about departing with a full heart and palate and arriving at the table eager for fresh experiences.

Therefore, whether you are cooking for one, a family, or entertaining friends, let the Come Hungry Cookbook be your guide to easy, enjoyable, and delicious meals. Embrace the joy of cooking with these **41 recipes**, and let your kitchen be a place where flavor and simplicity coexist beautifully.

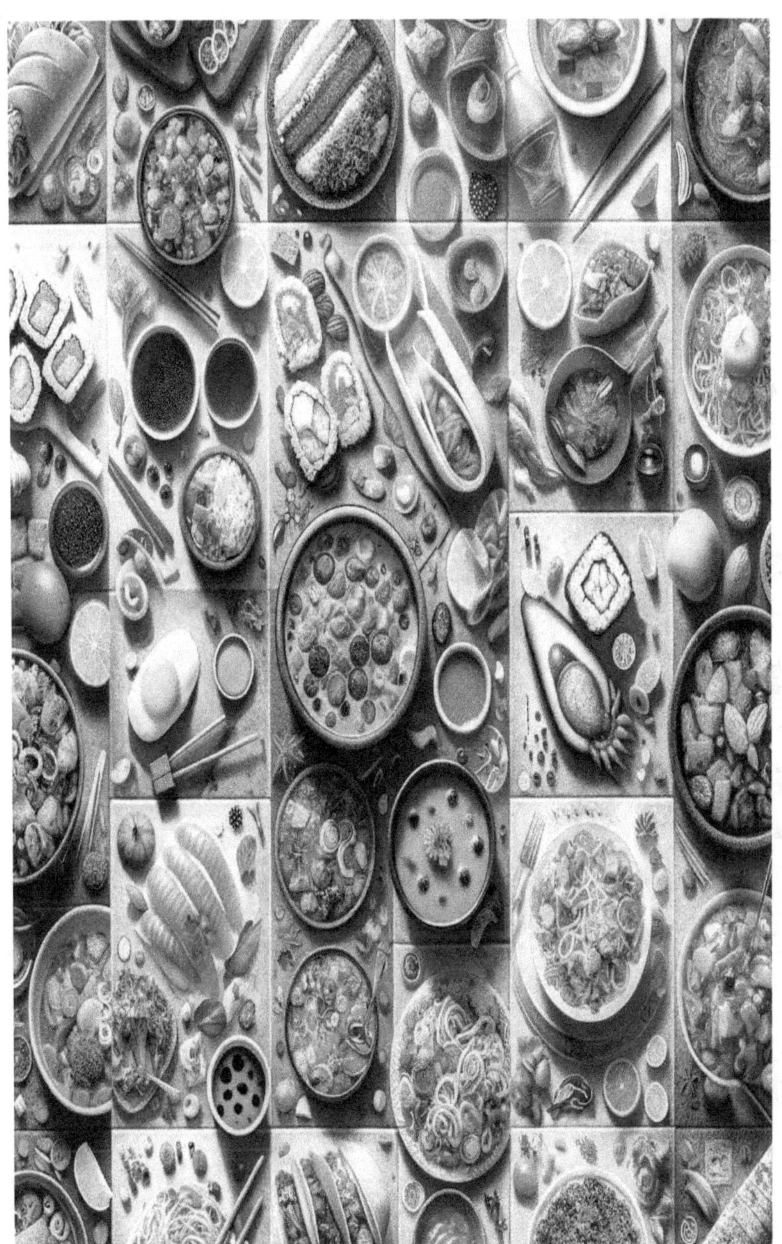

CHAPTER 1

Appetizing Starters

Introducing the first part of your culinary adventure with the Come Hungry Cookbook. We explore the world of delicious beginnings in Appetizing Starters, making sure every meal begins with a taste explosion and ease of preparation.

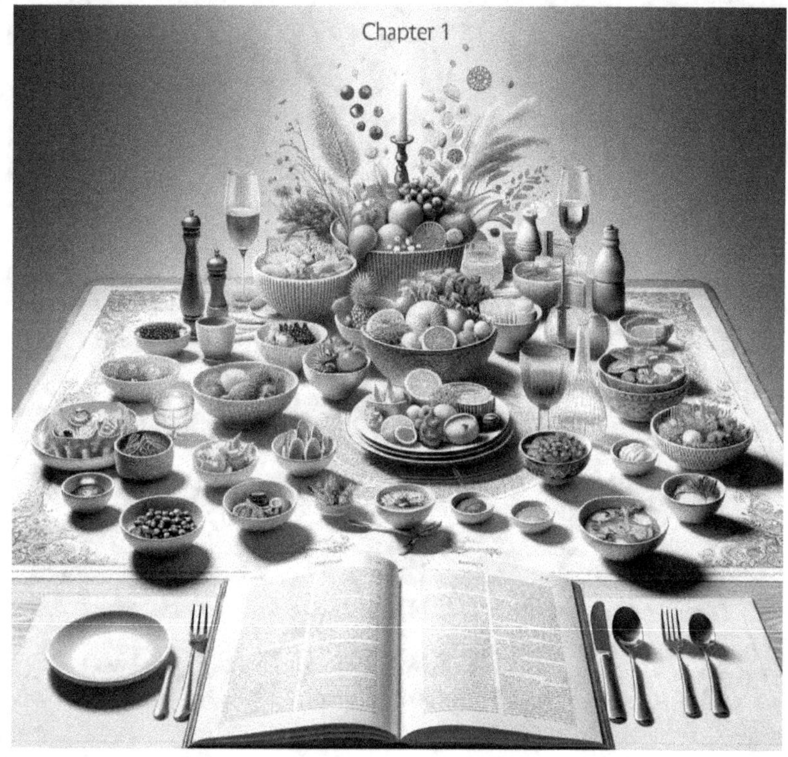

1. Sun-Dried Tomato and Feta Bruschetta

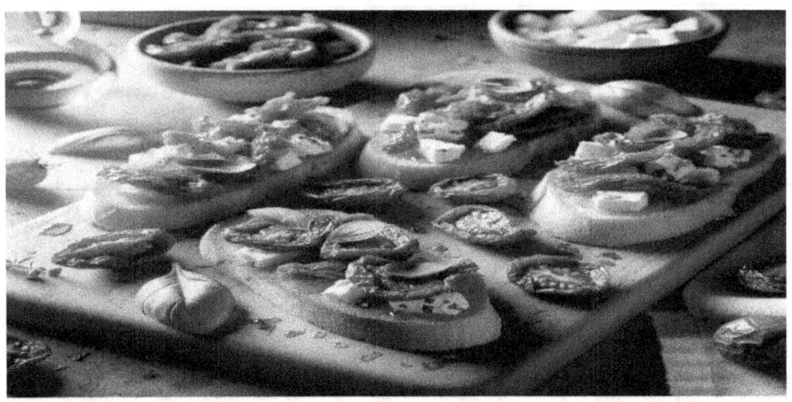

INGREDIENTS:

1 baguette, sliced into 1/2-inch pieces

1/2 cup sun-dried tomatoes in oil, drained and chopped

3/4 cup feta cheese, crumbled

1/4 cup fresh basil leaves, chopped

2 cloves garlic, minced

2 tablespoons olive oil

Salt and freshly ground black pepper, to taste

COOKING & PREP TIME

20 MINUTES

METHODS:

Preheat your oven to 375°F (190°C).

Arrange the baguette slices on a baking sheet and brush them lightly with olive oil. Toast in the oven for about 5 minutes, or until they are golden.

In a bowl, combine the chopped sun-dried tomatoes, crumbled feta cheese, minced garlic, and chopped basil. Season with salt and pepper to taste.

Spoon the tomato and feta mixture onto each toasted baguette slice. Serve immediately.

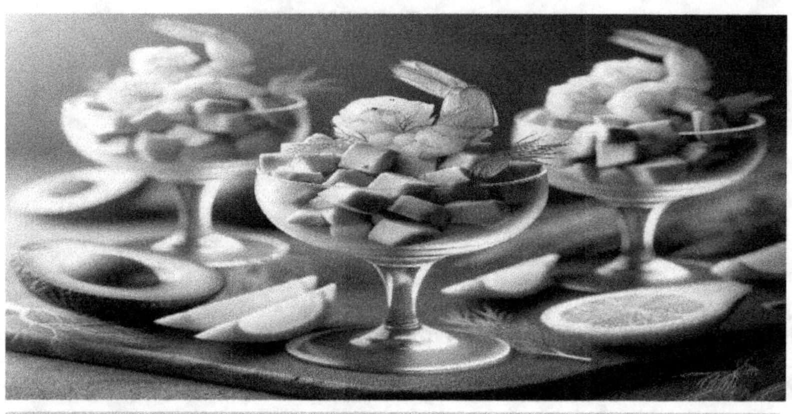

INGREDIENTS:

12 large shrimp, peeled and deveined

2 ripe avocados, halved and pitted

1/4 cup cocktail sauce

1-tablespoon fresh lime juice

1/2 teaspoon smoked paprika

Salt and pepper to taste

6 small lettuce leaves (for serving)

Optional: Fresh cilantro or parsley for garnish

METHODS:

1. Bring a pot of salted water to a boil.

2. Add the shrimp and cook for 2-3 minutes or until they are pink and opaque. Drain and set aside to cool.

3. In a bowl, mash the avocado with the lime juice, smoked paprika, salt, and pepper until smooth.

4. Arrange the lettuce leaves in six serving cups or small dishes.

5. Divide the mashed avocado evenly among the cups, placing it on top of the lettuce.

6. Place two shrimp in each cup and top each with a dollop of cocktail sauce.

7. Garnish with fresh cilantro or parsley if desired.

8. Serve immediately.

COOKING & PREP TIME

25 MINUTES

3. Spiced Chickpea and Cucumber Bites

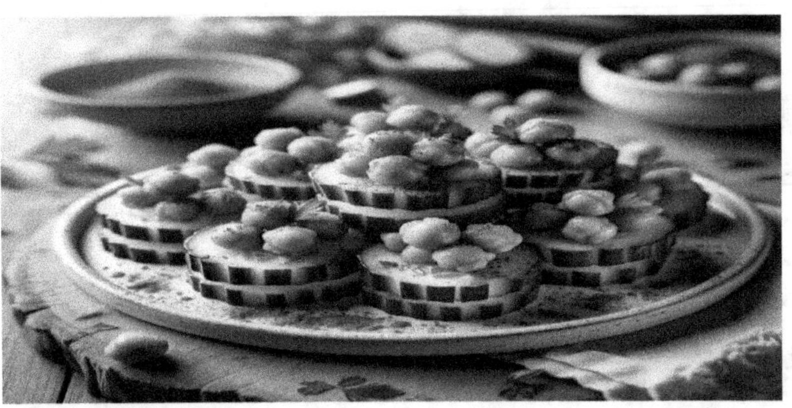

INGREDIENTS:	METHODS:

1 can (15 oz.) chickpeas, drained and rinsed

1 large cucumber, sliced into rounds

1-tablespoon olive oil

1-teaspoon ground cumin

1/2 teaspoon smoked paprika

1/4 teaspoon garlic powder

Salt and pepper to taste

Fresh parsley or cilantro, finely chopped, for garnish

1. In a bowl, toss the chickpeas with olive oil, cumin, smoked paprika, garlic powder, salt, and pepper until well coated.

2. Let the chickpeas marinate for 10 minutes to absorb the flavors.

3. Place a few chickpeas on top of each cucumber slice, pressing gently to ensure they stay in place.

4. Garnish each bite with a sprinkle of chopped parsley or cilantro.

5. Serve immediately, or chill in the refrigerator for a refreshing snack.

PREP TIME

15 MINUTES

4. Mini Caprese Skewers

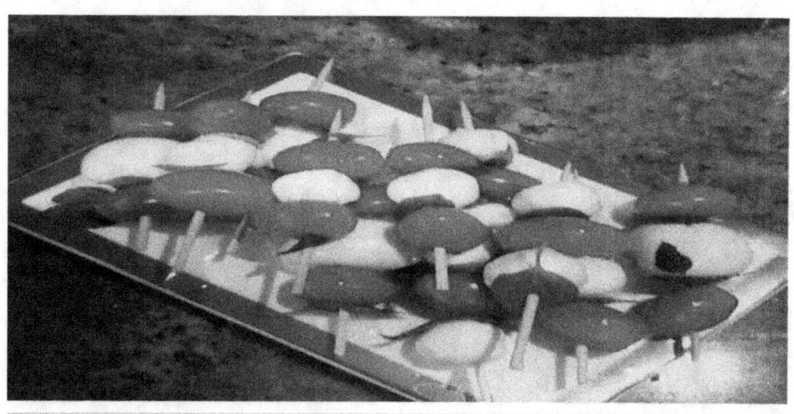

INGREDIENTS:	METHODS:

24 cherry tomatoes

12 mini mozzarella balls (bocconcini), halved

24 fresh basil leaves

12 toothpicks or small skewers

2 tablespoons extra virgin olive oil

1-tablespoon balsamic glaze (optional)

Salt and pepper to taste

1. Wash the cherry tomatoes and basil leaves and pat them dry.

2. Thread a tomato, a basil leaf, and a half mozzarella ball onto each toothpick. Repeat the process so that each skewer has two sets of tomato, basil, and mozzarella.

3. Arrange the skewers on a serving platter.

4. Drizzle with olive oil and balsamic glaze, if using.

5. Sprinkle with a pinch of salt and pepper to taste.

6. Serve immediately, or refrigerate until ready to serve.

PREP TIME

10 MINUTES

CHAPTER 2

Tantalizing Toasts

In this chapter of the "Come Hungry Cookbook," we explore the delicious and adaptable world of toasts, which are ideal for any time of day. We honor the simplicity of toasts and the countless options they present, regardless of how grandiose they are.

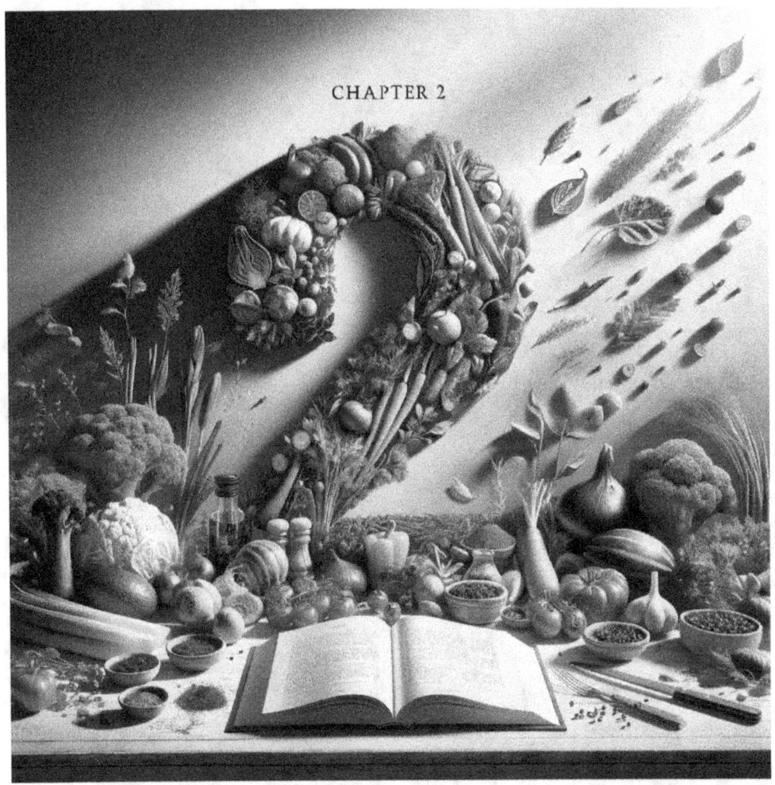

5. Classic Avocado and Poached Egg Toast

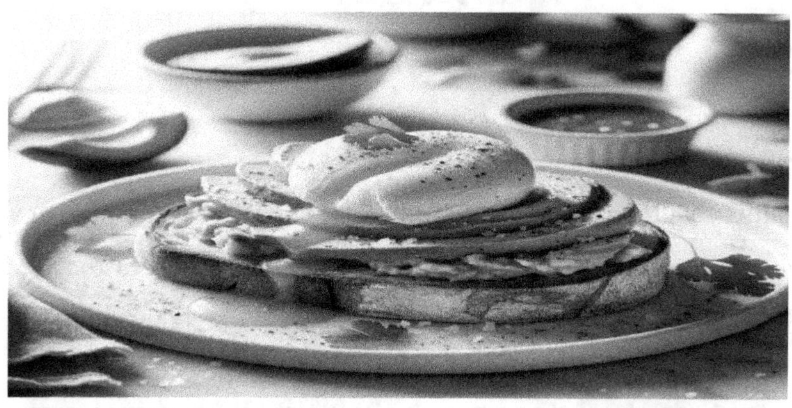

INGREDIENTS:

2 slices of whole-grain bread

1 ripe avocado

2 eggs

1-tablespoon white vinegar (for poaching eggs)

Salt and pepper to taste

Optional: Olive oil, red pepper flakes, fresh herbs (like parsley or chives) for garnish

COOKING & PREP TIME

15 MINUTES

METHODS:

1. Poach the Eggs:

Bring a pot of water to a gentle simmer and add the white vinegar.

Crack each egg into a small bowl and gently slide it into the simmering water.

Poach the eggs for about 3-4 minutes, or until the whites are set but the yolks are still runny.

2. Prepare the Avocado Toast:

Toast the bread slices to your desired level of crispness.

Halve the avocado, remove the pit, and scoop the flesh into a bowl.

Mash the avocado with a fork and season with salt and pepper.

Spread the mashed avocado evenly over the toasted bread slices.

3. Assemble:

Place a poached egg on top of each avocado toast.

Season with more salt and pepper, and add any optional garnishes like a drizzle of olive oil, red pepper flakes, or chopped fresh herbs.

6. Ricotta and Honeyed Peaches Toast

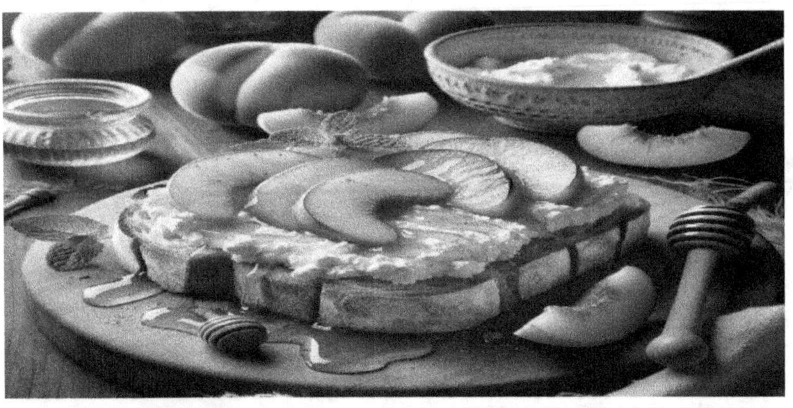

INGREDIENTS:	METHODS:

INGREDIENTS:

2 slices of whole-grain bread

1/2 cup ricotta cheese

1 ripe peach, sliced

2 tablespoons honey

Optional: A pinch of cinnamon or fresh mint for garnish

METHODS:

1. Toast the bread slices to your desired level of crispness.

2. Spread a generous layer of ricotta cheese on each slice of toast.

3. Arrange the peach slices over the ricotta.

4. Drizzle honey over the peaches.

5. If desired, sprinkle a pinch of cinnamon or add a few leaves of fresh mint for an extra burst of flavor and presentation.

6. Serve immediately and enjoy!

COOKING & PREP TIME

15 MINUTES

7. Smoked Salmon and Cream Cheese Toast

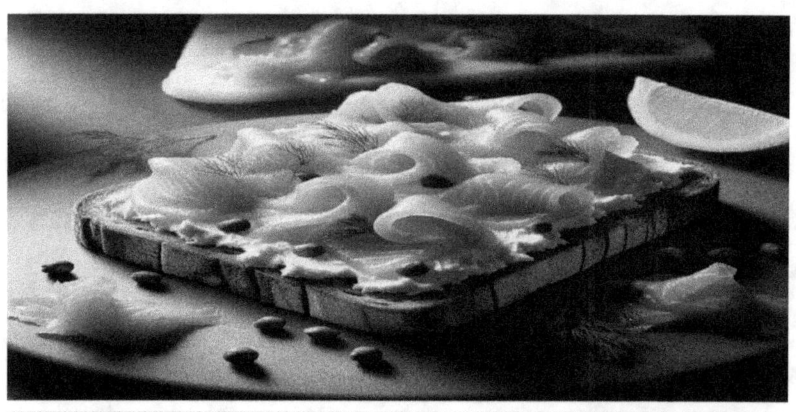

INGREDIENTS:

2 slices of whole-grain bread

4 oz. smoked salmon

2 tablespoons cream cheese

1 tablespoon capers (optional)

1 teaspoon fresh dill, chopped

Freshly ground black pepper, to taste

Lemon wedges for serving

COOKING & PREP TIME

15 MINUTES

METHODS:

1. Toast the bread slices to your desired level of crispness.

2. Spread each slice of toast with cream cheese.

3. Place smoked salmon evenly on top of the cream cheese.

4. Sprinkle capers (if using) and fresh dill over the salmon.

5. Add freshly ground black pepper to taste.

6. Serve with a lemon wedge on the side.

8. Roasted Tomato and Basil Pesto Toast

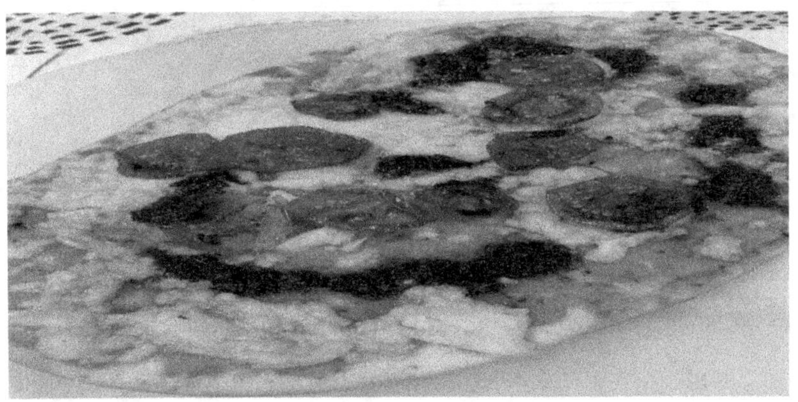

INGREDIENTS:	METHODS:

INGREDIENTS:

4 large tomatoes, sliced

2 slices of whole-grain bread

4 tablespoons basil pesto

2 teaspoons olive oil

Salt and pepper to taste

Optional: Shavings of Parmesan cheese or fresh basil leaves for garnish

METHODS:

1. Roast the Tomatoes:

Preheat the oven to 375°F (190°C).

Place the tomato slices on a baking sheet, drizzle with olive oil, and season with salt and pepper.

Roast in the oven for about 20 minutes or until the tomatoes are tender and slightly caramelized.

2. Prepare the Toast:

Toast the bread slices to your desired level of crispness.

3. Assemble the Toast:

Spread each slice of toast with 2 tablespoons of basil pesto.

Arrange the roasted tomatoes on top of the pesto.

If desired, garnish with Parmesan cheese shavings or fresh basil leaves.

Serve immediately and enjoy!

COOKING & PREP TIME

35 MINUTES

CHAPTER 3

Fresh and Flavorful Salads

Here in the Come Hungry Cookbook, we explore the colorful world of salads. These are star performers, full of flavors, textures, and colors, not just side dishes. These salads are meant to be both filling and enjoyable, making them ideal for anyone on a diet or just someone searching for something new and great to eat.

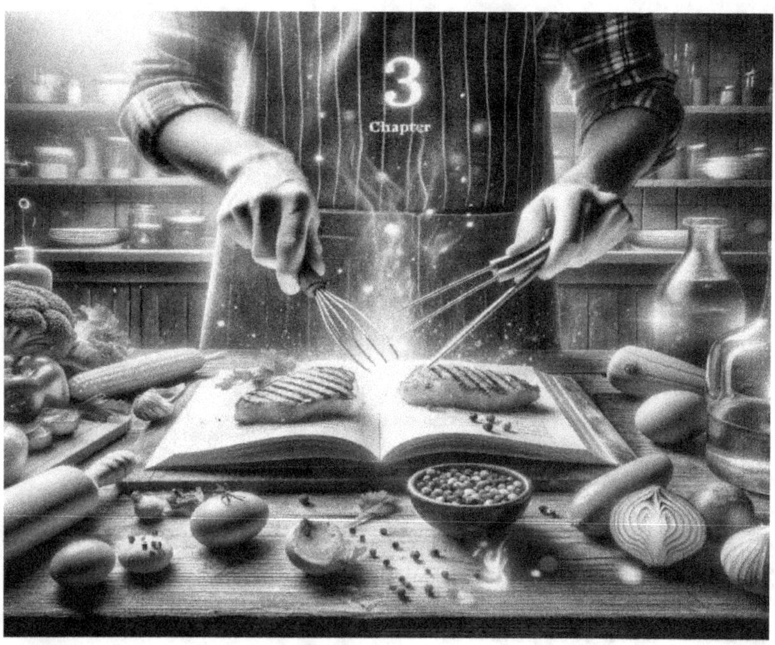

9. Crispy Chickpea and Quinoa Salad

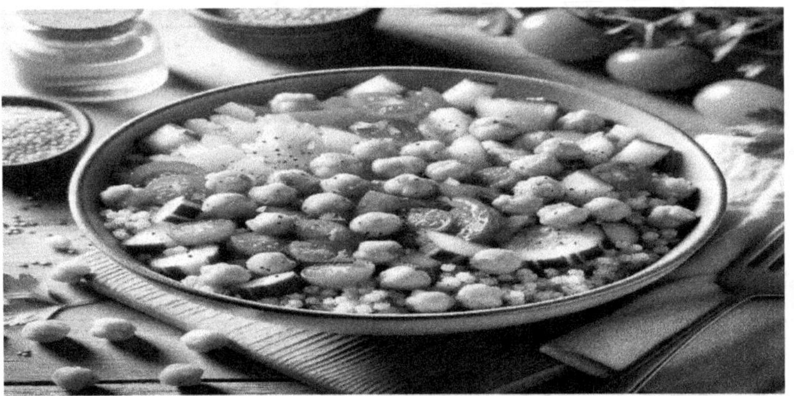

INGREDIENTS:

1 cup quinoa, rinsed

1 can (15 oz.) chickpeas, drained, rinsed, and dried

1 cucumber, diced

1 bell pepper, diced

1/2 red onion, finely chopped

1/4 cup fresh parsley, chopped

3 tablespoons olive oil (divided)

2 tablespoons lemon juice

1-teaspoon ground cumin

Salt and pepper to taste

COOKING & PREP TIME

50 MINUTES

METHODS:

1. Cook Quinoa:

In a saucepan, bring 2 cups of water to a boil. Add quinoa, reduce heat to low, cover, and simmer for 15-20 minutes until quinoa is tender and water is absorbed.

Fluff with a fork and set aside to cool.

2. Roast Chickpeas:

Preheat the oven to 400°F (200°C).

Toss chickpeas with 1 tablespoon of olive oil, cumin, salt, and pepper.

Spread them on a baking sheet and roast for 20-30 minutes, or until crispy.

3. Prepare Salad:

In a large bowl, combine the cooked quinoa, roasted chickpeas, cucumber, bell pepper, red onion, and parsley.

4. Dressing:

Whisk together 2 tablespoons of olive oil with lemon juice. Season with salt and pepper.

Pour the dressing over the salad and toss to combine.

Serve immediately

10. Watermelon, Feta, and Mint Salad

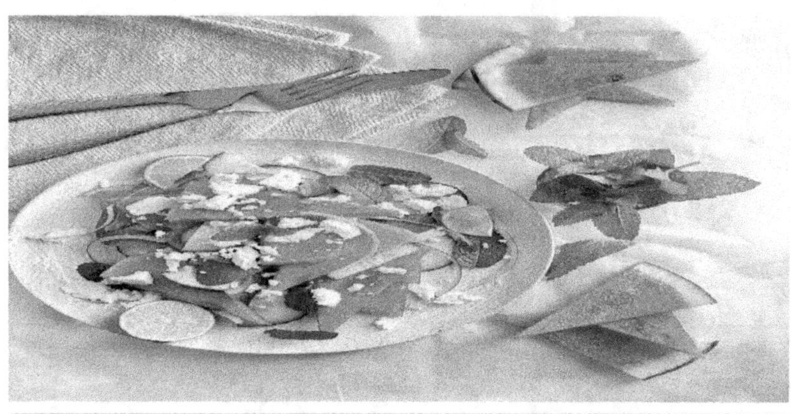

INGREDIENTS:	METHODS:

INGREDIENTS:

4 cups cubed watermelon

1 cup feta cheese, crumbled

1/4 cup fresh mint leaves, torn

2 tablespoons olive oil

1-tablespoon balsamic vinegar

Salt and pepper to taste

METHODS:

1. In a large bowl, gently combine the cubed watermelon, crumbled feta cheese, and torn mint leaves.

2. In a small bowl, whisk together the olive oil and balsamic vinegar. Season with a pinch of salt and pepper.

3. Drizzle the dressing over the watermelon mixture and toss gently to coat.

4. Serve the salad chilled or at room temperature.

PREP TIME

15 MINUTES

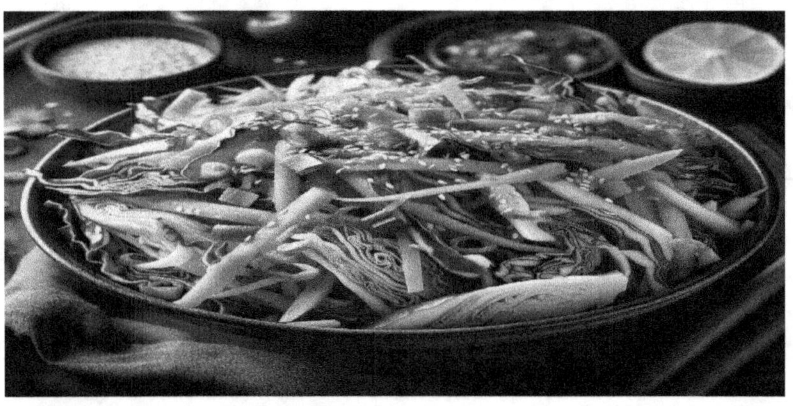

INGREDIENTS:

1. For the Slaw:

2 cups shredded cabbage (mix of red and green)

1 carrot, julienned

1 bell pepper, thinly sliced

1/2 cucumber, julienned

1/4 cup chopped green onions

1/4 cup chopped cilantro

2. For the Sesame Ginger Dressing:

3 tablespoons sesame oil

2 tablespoons rice vinegar

1-tablespoon soy sauce

1-tablespoon honey

1 teaspoon grated ginger

1 garlic clove, minced

Salt and pepper to taste

METHODS:

1. In a large bowl, combine the shredded cabbage, julienned carrot, sliced bell pepper, julienned cucumber, chopped green onions, and cilantro.

2. In a small bowl, whisk together the sesame oil, rice vinegar, soy sauce, honey, grated ginger, and minced garlic. Season with salt and pepper to taste.

3. Pour the dressing over the slaw and toss well to combine.

4. Let the slaw sit for about 10 minutes to allow the flavors to meld.

5. Garnish with sesame seeds and chopped peanuts if desired.

6. Serve as a refreshing side dish or a light meal.

PREP TIME

20 MINUTES

12. Roasted Beet and Goat Cheese Salad

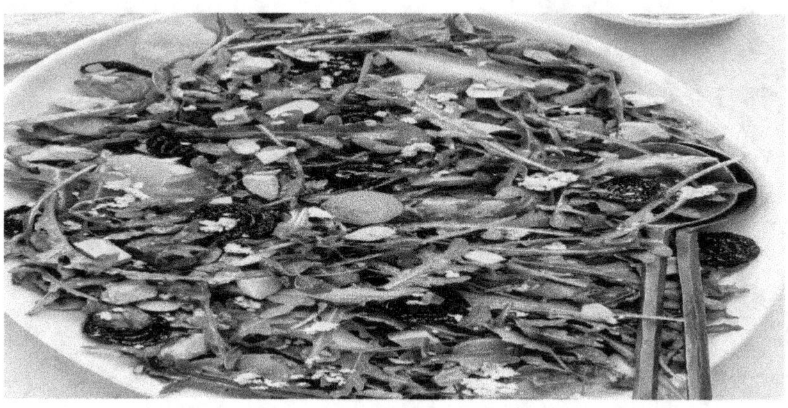

INGREDIENTS:

4 medium beets, trimmed and scrubbed

6 cups mixed greens (like arugula and spinach)

1/2 cup goat cheese, crumbled

1/4 cup walnuts, toasted and chopped

3 tablespoons olive oil

1-tablespoon balsamic vinegar

Salt and pepper to taste

Optional: Fresh herbs (such as thyme or parsley) for garnish

COOKING & PREP TIME

60 MINUTES

METHODS:

1. Roast Beets:

Preheat the oven to 400°F (200°C).

Wrap each beet individually in foil and place them on a baking sheet.

Roast in the oven for about 45 minutes or until tender. Once cooled, peel and slice the beets.

2. Prepare the Salad:

In a large bowl, place the mixed greens.

Add the sliced roasted beets and crumbled goat cheese.

Sprinkle the toasted walnuts over the salad.

3. Dressing:

In a small bowl, whisk together olive oil, balsamic vinegar, salt, and pepper.

Drizzle the dressing over the salad and gently toss to combine.

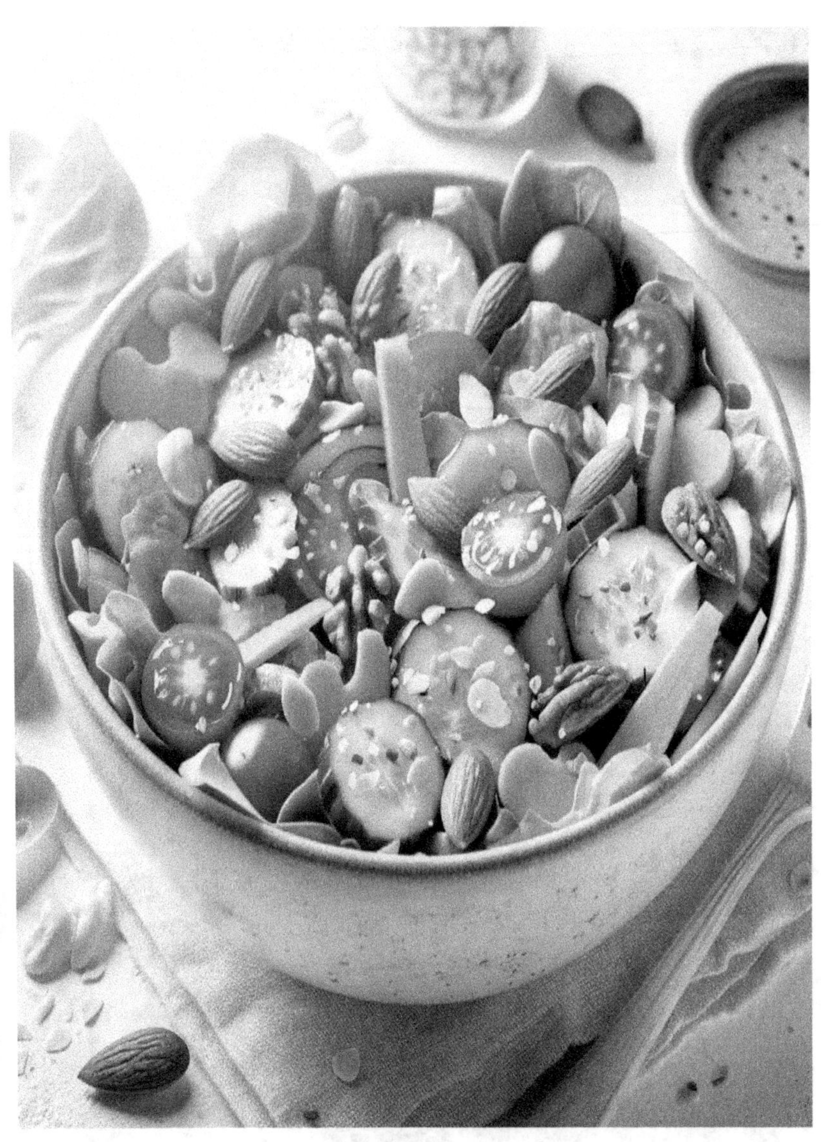

CHAPTER 4

Hearty Grain Salads

In this chapter from the "Come Hungry Cookbook," we delve into the healthy and filling realm of grain salads. These meals are ideal for each meal of the day because they are not only nutrient-dense but also bursting with a variety of flavors and textures.

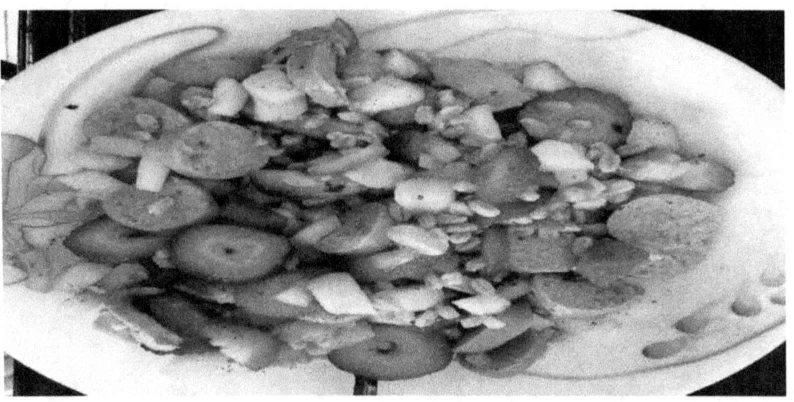

INGREDIENTS:

1 cup farro, rinsed

2 cups water or vegetable broth

1 cucumber, diced

1 bell pepper, diced

1/2 red onion, finely chopped

1/2 cup cherry tomatoes, halved

1/2 cup Kalamata olives, pitted and sliced

1/2 cup feta cheese, crumbled

1/4 cup fresh parsley, chopped

3 tablespoons olive oil

2 tablespoons red wine vinegar

1 garlic clove, minced

Salt and pepper to taste

COOKING & PREP TIME

50 MINUTES

METHODS:

1. Cook Farro:

In a saucepan, bring the water or vegetable broth to a boil. Add farro, reduce the heat to low, cover, and simmer for about 25-30 minutes until the farro is tender and the liquid is absorbed.

Drain any excess liquid and let the farro cool.

2. Prepare the Salad:

In a large bowl, combine the cooled farro, diced cucumber, bell pepper, red onion, cherry tomatoes, Kalamata olives, and crumbled feta cheese.

3. Dressing:

In a small bowl, whisk together olive oil, red wine vinegar, minced garlic, salt, and pepper.

Pour the dressing over the salad and toss to combine.

Stir in the chopped parsley.

Serve the salad at room temperature or chilled.

14. Spicy Southwest Quinoa Salad

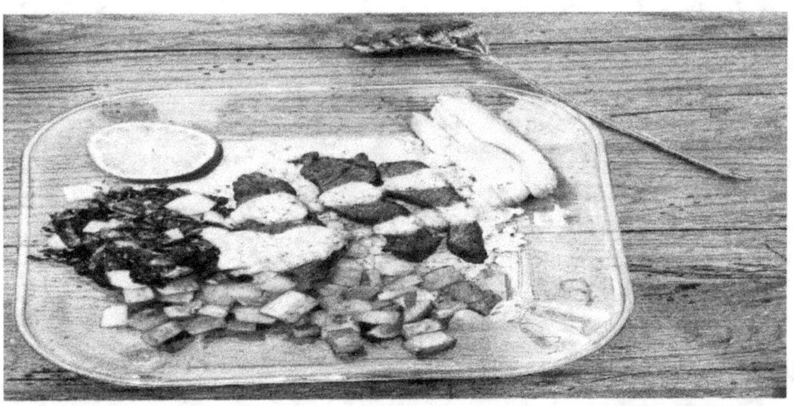

INGREDIENTS:	METHODS:

INGREDIENTS:

1 cup quinoa, rinsed

2 cups water

1 can (15 oz.) black beans, drained and rinsed

1-cup corn kernels (fresh or frozen)

1 red bell pepper, diced

1/2 red onion, finely chopped

1/4 cup fresh cilantro, chopped

For the Dressing:

3 tablespoons olive oil

2 tablespoons lime juice

1-teaspoon ground cumin

1/2 teaspoon chili powder

1/4 teaspoon cayenne pepper

COOKING & PREP TIME

45 MINUTES

METHODS:

1. Cook Quinoa:

In a saucepan, bring the water to a boil. Add quinoa, reduce heat to low, cover, and simmer for about 15 minutes until the quinoa is tender and the water is absorbed.

Fluff with a fork and let it cool.

2. Prepare the Salad:

In a large bowl, combine the cooled quinoa, black beans, corn, red bell pepper, red onion, and cilantro.

3. Make the Dressing:

In a small bowl, whisk together olive oil, lime juice, cumin, chili powder, cayenne pepper, salt, and pepper.

Pour the dressing over the salad and toss to combine.

Serve the salad chilled.

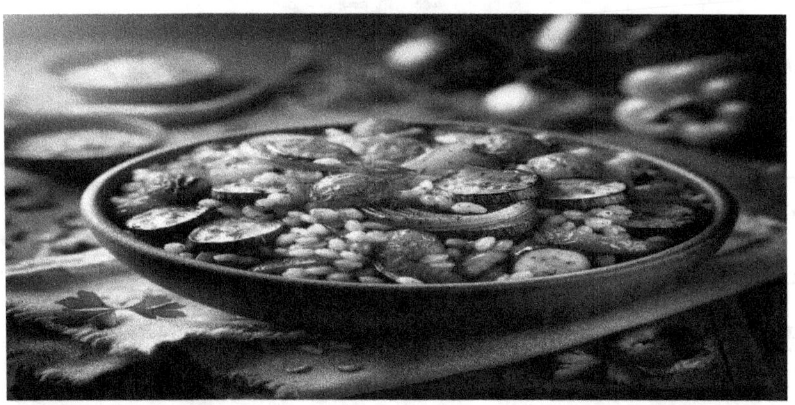

INGREDIENTS:

1-cup pearl barley

2 cups vegetable broth

1 zucchini, chopped

1 red bell pepper, chopped

1 yellow bell pepper, chopped

1 red onion, chopped

2 carrots, chopped

3 tablespoons olive oil

2 tablespoons balsamic vinegar

Salt and pepper to taste

COOKING & PREP TIME

55 MINUTES

METHODS:

1. Cook Barley:

In a saucepan, bring the vegetable broth to a boil. Add barley, reduce the heat to low, cover, and simmer for about 30-40 minutes until the barley is tender and the liquid is absorbed.

Fluff with a fork and set aside to cool slightly.

2. Roast Vegetables:

Preheat the oven to 400°F (200°C).

Toss the chopped vegetables with 2 tablespoons of olive oil, salt, and pepper.

Spread them on a baking sheet and roast for about 20-25 minutes, or until they are tender and caramelized.

3. Prepare the Salad:

In a large bowl, combine the warm barley and roasted vegetables.

4. Dressing:

Whisk together 1 tablespoon of olive oil with balsamic vinegar. Season with salt and pepper.

Drizzle the dressing over the salad and toss to combine.

Garnish with fresh herbs if desired.

Serve warm or at room temperature.

Quick & Savory Dinners

In the "Come Hungry Cookbook," this chapter is devoted to Easy & Tasty Dinner Recipes. All of these dishes are designed to maximize taste, heartiness, and warmth at your dinner table while requiring the least amount of prep work. Even on the busiest of days, you may enjoy a fulfilling lunch thanks to the careful preparation of each dish.

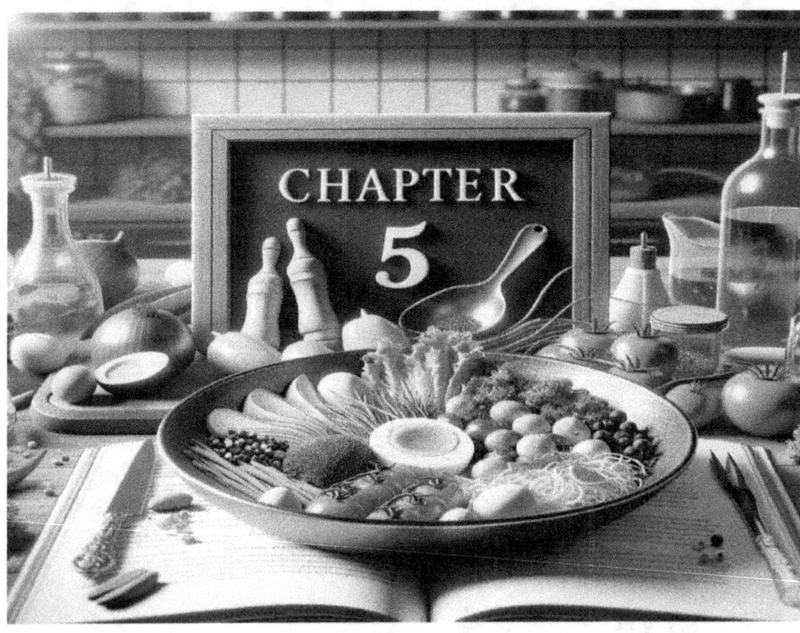

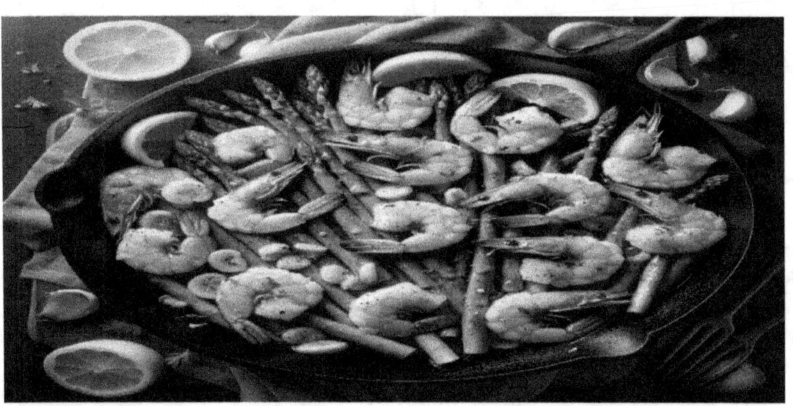

INGREDIENTS:

1 lb. large shrimp, peeled and deveined

1 bunch of asparagus, ends trimmed and cut into thirds

3 tablespoons olive oil

4 cloves garlic, minced

1 lemon, juiced and zested

Salt and pepper, to taste

Red pepper flakes (optional, for heat)

2 tablespoons fresh parsley, chopped (for garnish)

COOKING & PREP TIME

20 MINUTES

METHODS:

1. Preheat & Prepare: Preheat your skillet over medium-high heat. While the skillet is heating, toss the shrimp and asparagus in olive oil, garlic, lemon zest, and seasonings.

2. Cook Asparagus: Place the asparagus in the skillet and cook for about 4-5 minutes, or until it becomes tender-crisp. Remove the asparagus from the skillet and set aside.

3. Cook Shrimp: In the same skillet, add the shrimp. Cook for about 2 minutes on each side or until they turn pink and opaque. Be careful not to overcook.

4. Combine & Finish: Return the asparagus to the skillet with the shrimp. Drizzle with lemon juice and toss to combine. Cook for an additional minute to reheat the asparagus.

5. Garnish & Serve: Garnish with fresh parsley and additional lemon slices if desired. Serve immediately.

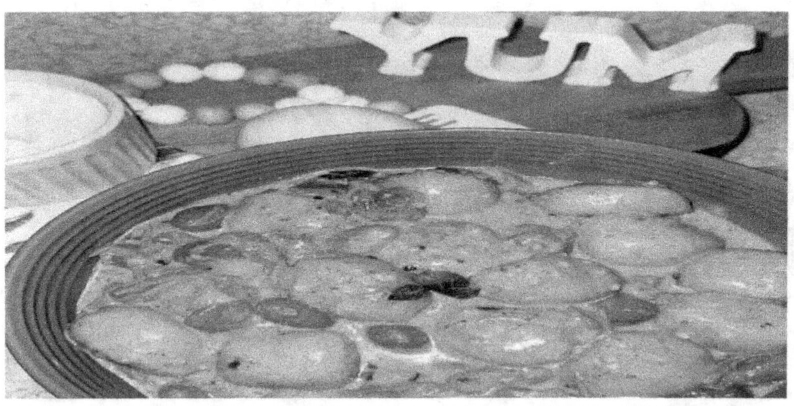

INGREDIENTS:

8 ounces pasta (like fettuccine, penne, or spaghetti)

2 tablespoons olive oil

1 small onion, finely chopped

3 cloves garlic, minced

1 can (14 ounces) crushed tomatoes

1/2 cup heavy cream or full-fat coconut milk for a vegan option

1/4 cup freshly grated Parmesan cheese (omit for vegan version)

1/2 cup fresh basil leaves, chopped

Salt and pepper, to taste

Red pepper flakes (optional, for heat)

Additional basil leaves for garnish

COOKING & PREP TIME

30 MINUTES

METHODS:

1. Cook Pasta: Cook the pasta according to package instructions until al dente. Drain and set aside, reserving some pasta water.

2. Sauté Aromatics: In a large skillet, heat olive oil over medium heat. Add onion and garlic, sautéing until the onion is translucent and fragrant.

3. Add Tomatoes & Simmer: Stir in crushed tomatoes. Bring to a simmer and cook for about 10 minutes, or until the sauce starts to thicken.

4. Make Creamy Sauce: Lower the heat and stir in heavy cream and Parmesan cheese (if using). Cook for an additional 2-3 minutes, until the sauce is creamy and heated through.

5. Combine Pasta & Sauce: Add the cooked pasta to the sauce, tossing to coat evenly. If the sauce is too thick, add a little reserved pasta water to reach your desired consistency.

6. Season & Garnish: Stir in chopped basil, and season with salt, pepper, and red pepper flakes if desired. Garnish with additional basil leaves.

7. Serve: Serve hot, offering extra Parmesan cheese on the side if desired.

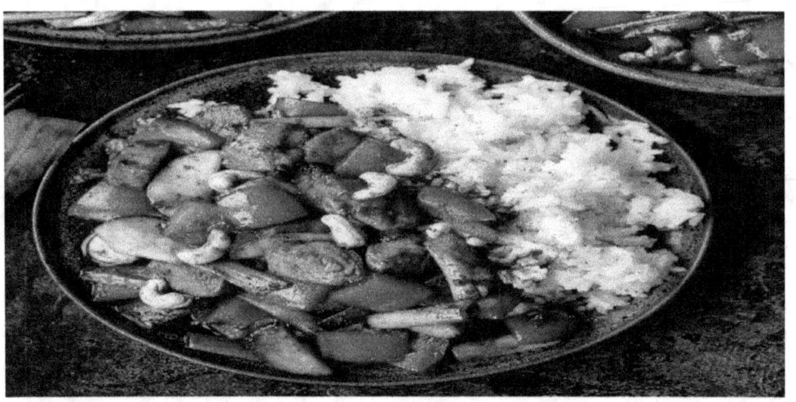

INGREDIENTS:

1 lb. chicken breast, thinly sliced

2 tablespoons soy sauce

1-tablespoon sesame oil

1-tablespoon cornstarch

2 tablespoons vegetable oil

1 red bell pepper, sliced

1-cup broccoli florets

1 carrot, thinly sliced

2 cloves garlic, minced

1 inch ginger, grated

2 tablespoons hoisin sauce

1 tablespoon chili sauce (adjust to taste)

Salt and pepper, to taste

COOKING & PREP TIME

25 MINUTES

METHODS:

1. Marinate Chicken: In a bowl, combine sliced chicken, soy sauce, sesame oil, and cornstarch. Let it marinate for at least 10 minutes.

2. Cook Chicken: Heat 1 tablespoon of vegetable oil in a large skillet or wok over medium-high heat. Add the chicken in batches, cooking until browned and cooked through. Remove chicken and set aside.

3. Stir-Fry Vegetables: Add the remaining tablespoon of oil to the skillet. Add bell pepper, broccoli, and carrot, stir-frying for about 3-4 minutes until they are tender-crisp.

4. Add Aromatics: Include garlic and ginger to the vegetables, cooking for another minute until fragrant.

5. Combine with Sauce: Return the chicken to the skillet. Add hoisin sauce and chili sauce, tossing everything together to coat well. Cook for 1-2 minutes more.

6. Season & Serve: Season with salt and pepper to taste. Garnish with green onions and sesame seeds.

7. Serve Hot: Serve immediately, optionally with rice or noodles.

19. Vegetarian Stuffed Peppers

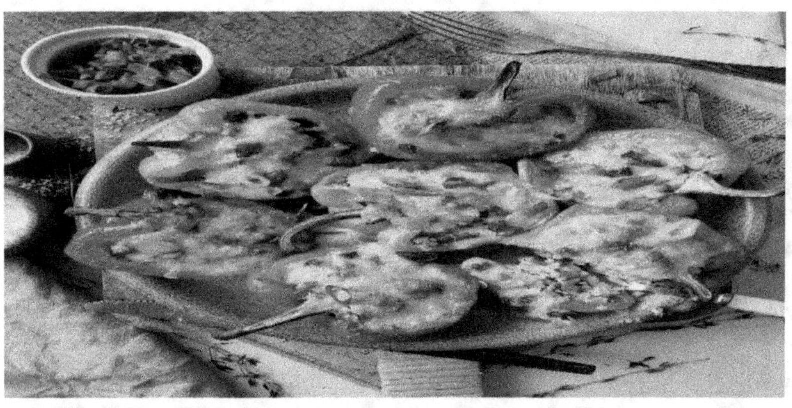

INGREDIENTS:	METHODS:

INGREDIENTS:

4 large bell peppers, tops cut off and seeds removed

1 cup cooked quinoa or rice

1 can (15 ounces) black beans, rinsed and drained

1-cup corn kernels (fresh, canned, or frozen)

1/2 cup diced tomatoes

1/2 cup onion, finely chopped

2 cloves garlic, minced

1-teaspoon cumin

1-teaspoon paprika

Salt and pepper, to taste

1 cup shredded cheddar or Monterey Jack cheese (use vegan cheese for a vegan option)

METHODS:

1. Preheat Oven: Preheat the oven to 375°F (190°C).

2. Prepare Peppers: Arrange the bell peppers in a baking dish. If necessary, slightly trim the bottoms to help them stand upright.

3. Make Filling: In a large bowl, mix the cooked quinoa or rice, black beans, corn, diced tomatoes, onion, garlic, cumin, paprika, salt, and pepper.

4. Stuff Peppers: Spoon the filling into each bell pepper cavity and press down gently to pack it in.

5. Bake: Cover the baking dish with aluminium foil and bake for about 25 minutes.

6. Add Cheese: Remove the foil, top each pepper with cheese, and bake uncovered for an additional 5 minutes, or until the cheese is melted and bubbly.

COOKING & PREP TIME

45 MINUTES

20. Pan-seared salmon with Dill Sauce

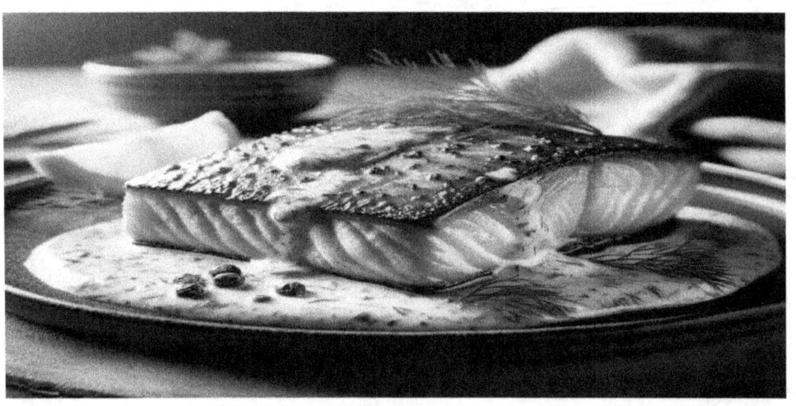

INGREDIENTS:

4 salmon fillets (about 6 ounces each)

2 tablespoons olive oil

Salt and pepper, to taste

1/2 cup sour cream (use a dairy-free alternative for a vegan option)

2 tablespoons fresh dill, chopped

1-tablespoon lemon juice

1-teaspoon lemon zest

1 clove garlic, minced

COOKING & PREP TIME

25 MINUTES

METHODS:

1. Prepare Salmon: Season the salmon fillets with salt and pepper on both sides.

2. Cook Salmon: Heat olive oil in a large skillet over medium-high heat. Place the salmon fillets in the skillet, skin-side down, and cook for about 6-7 minutes. Flip the fillets and cook for an additional 6-7 minutes, or until the salmon is cooked through and easily flakes with a fork.

3. Make Dill Sauce: While the salmon is cooking, mix sour cream, chopped dill, lemon juice, lemon zest, and minced garlic in a small bowl. Season with salt and pepper to taste.

4. Serve: Place the cooked salmon on plates, drizzle with the dill sauce, and garnish with extra dill and lemon slices if desired.

5. Enjoy: Serve immediately, ideally with a side of vegetables or a salad.

CHAPTER 6

Versatile Sides

Within the sixth chapter of the "Come Hungry Cookbook," we explore the realm of Versatile Sides. These recipes are meant to go well with your main courses and give your meals more flavor and depth. These sides, which range from grains to veggies, are not only great as side dishes but as stand-alone stars.

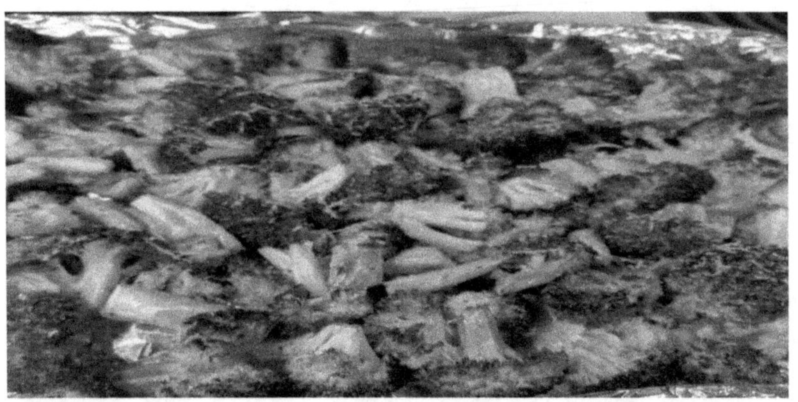

INGREDIENTS:

1 large head of broccoli, cut into florets

3 tablespoons olive oil

4 cloves garlic, minced

1/2 cup grated Parmesan cheese

Salt and pepper, to taste

Lemon zest or juice (optional, for added zest)

Red pepper flakes (optional, for heat)

COOKING & PREP TIME

30 MINUTES

METHODS:

1. Preheat Oven: Preheat your oven to 400°F (200°C).

2. Prepare Broccoli: In a large bowl, toss the broccoli florets with olive oil, minced garlic, and a sprinkle of salt and pepper.

3. Roast Broccoli: Spread the broccoli in a single layer on a baking sheet. Roast in the preheated oven for 15-20 minutes, or until the broccoli is tender and the edges are crispy.

4. Add Parmesan: Once the broccoli is out of the oven, immediately sprinkle grated Parmesan cheese over the hot broccoli. Toss to coat evenly.

5. Season & Serve: If desired, add lemon zest or juice, and red pepper flakes for an extra zing. Serve warm as a side dish.

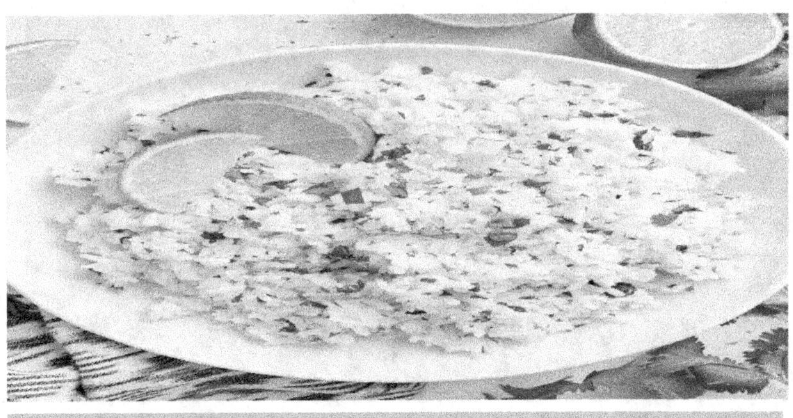

INGREDIENTS:

1 cup long-grain white rice

2 cups water

1 tablespoon olive oil

Zest of 1 lime

Juice of 1 lime

1/4 cup fresh cilantro, chopped

Salt, to taste

METHODS:

1. Cook Rice: In a medium saucepan, combine rice, water, and a pinch of salt. Bring to a boil over high heat. Once boiling, reduce the heat to low, cover, and simmer for about 18-20 minutes, or until the water is absorbed and the rice is tender.

2. Flavor Rice: Remove the rice from the heat. Add olive oil, lime zest, and lime juice. Fluff the rice with a fork to mix in the flavors.

3. Add Cilantro: Stir in the fresh cilantro, and adjust salt to taste.

4. Serve: Serve the rice warm as a side dish to complement a variety of main courses.

COOKING & PREP TIME

30 MINUTES

23. Maple Glazed Carrots

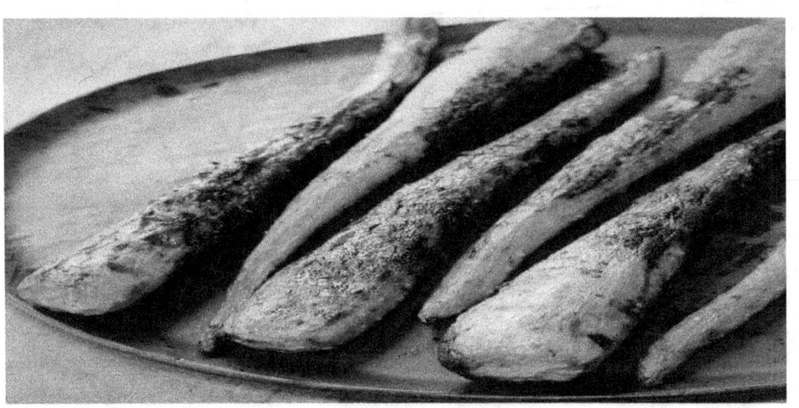

INGREDIENTS:

1 pound carrots, peeled and sliced diagonally

2 tablespoons butter (or olive oil for a vegan option)

3 tablespoons pure maple syrup

Salt and pepper, to taste

A pinch of ground cinnamon (optional)

Fresh parsley, chopped (for garnish)

COOKING & PREP TIME

35 MINUTES

METHODS:

1. Cook Carrots: In a large skillet, add the carrots and just enough water to cover them. Bring to a boil, then reduce heat and simmer until the carrots are tender about 10-15 minutes. 2. 2. Drain any remaining water.

3. Glaze Carrots: In the same skillet, melt butter over medium heat. Stir in the maple syrup, salt, pepper, and optional cinnamon. Add the cooked carrots and toss to coat evenly with the glaze.

4. Caramelize: Continue to cook, stirring occasionally, for about 5-10 minutes, or until the carrots are nicely glazed and slightly caramelized.

5. Garnish & Serve: Remove from heat. Garnish with chopped parsley before serving.

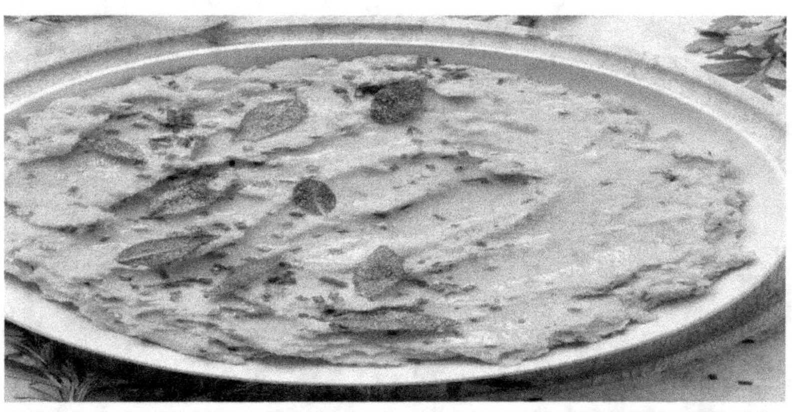

INGREDIENTS:

2 pounds sweet potatoes, peeled and cut into chunks

3 tablespoons butter (or olive oil for a vegan option)

2 cloves garlic, minced

1/4 cup milk (or almond milk for a vegan option)

Salt and pepper, to taste

1/4 teaspoon ground cinnamon

1/4 teaspoon smoked paprika

COOKING & PREP TIME

40 MINUTES

METHODS:

1. Boil Sweet Potatoes: Place sweet potato chunks in a large pot and cover with water. Bring to a boil, then reduce heat and simmer for 20-25 minutes, or until the potatoes are very tender.

2. Mash Potatoes: Drain the sweet potatoes and return them to the pot. Add butter, minced garlic, milk, salt, pepper, cinnamon, and smoked paprika. Mash until smooth and well combined. 3. 3. Adjust seasoning to taste.

4. Garnish & Serve: Garnish with fresh herbs and serve warm as a side dish.

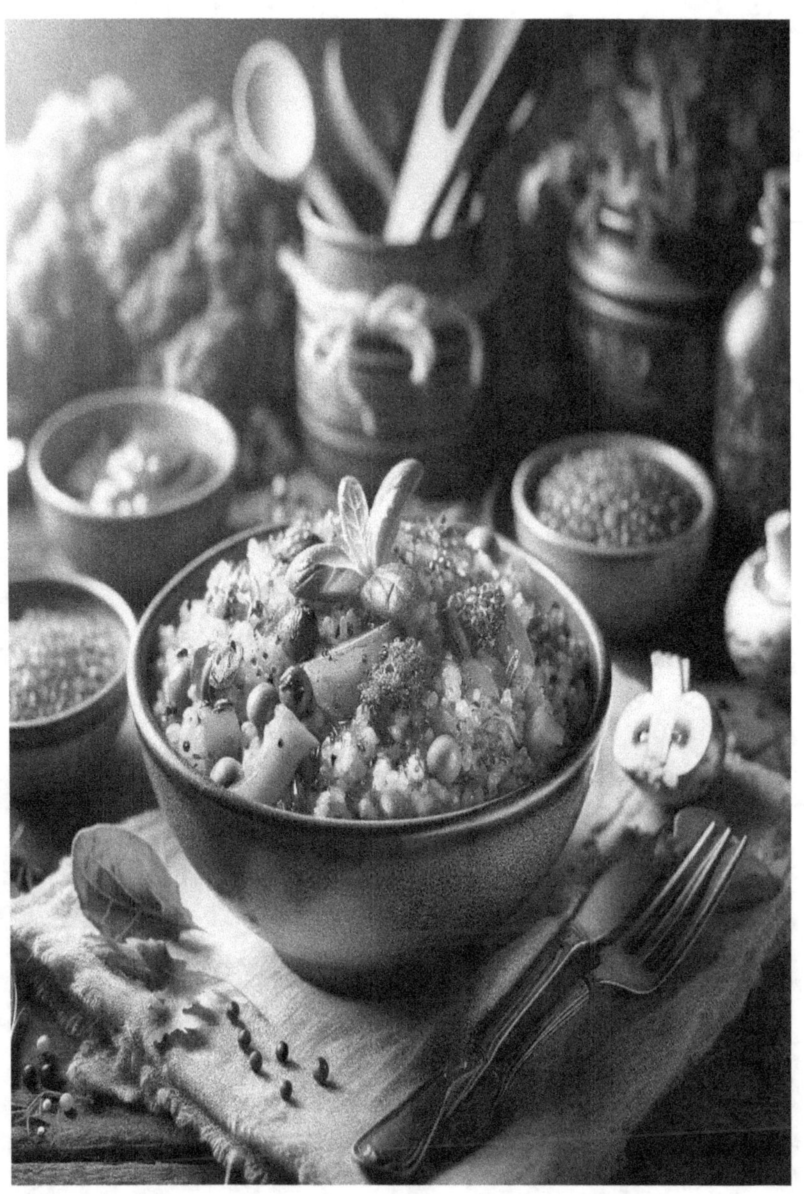

CHAPTER 7

Homemade Dressings

In the "Come Hungry Cookbook," we delve into the craft of homemade dressings in the seventh chapter. These are the culinary world's secret weapons, able to elevate simple salads, grains, and entrees to astonishing culinary feats.

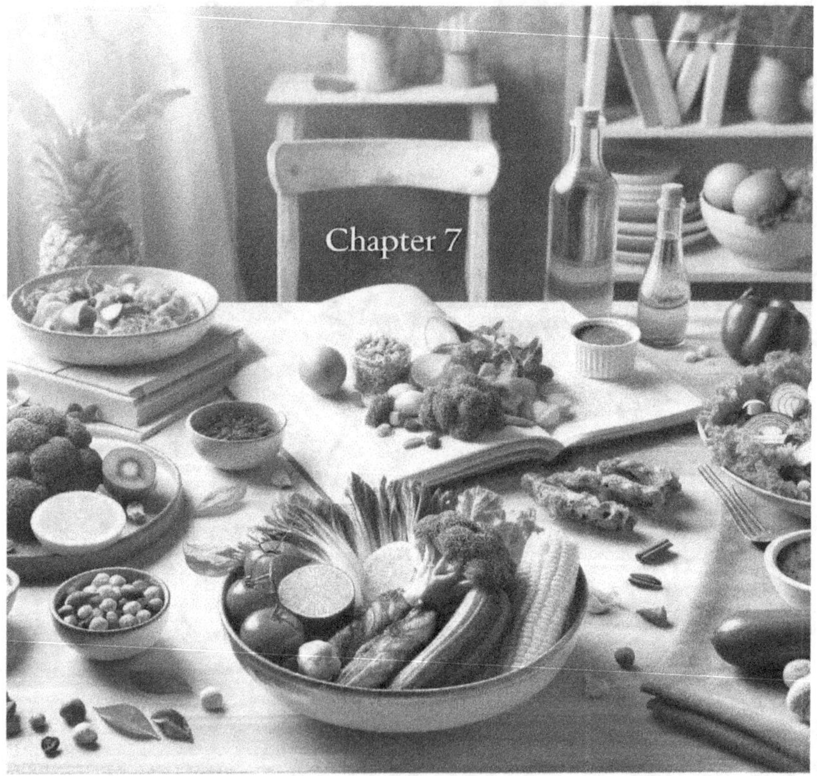

25. Classic Balsamic Vinaigrette

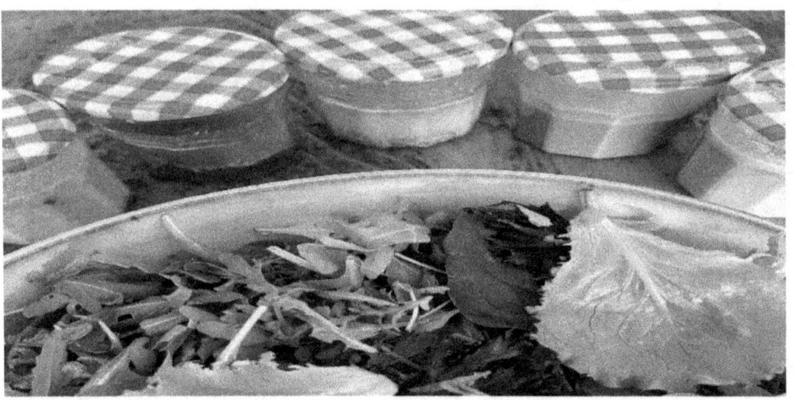

INGREDIENTS:

1/2 cup balsamic vinegar

1/2 cup extra virgin olive oil

1 clove garlic, minced

1 teaspoon Dijon mustard

1 teaspoon honey (optional, for added sweetness)

Salt and pepper, to taste

METHODS:

1. Combine Ingredients: In a small bowl, whisk together the balsamic vinegar, olive oil, minced garlic, Dijon mustard, and honey (if using).

2. Season: Season with salt and pepper to taste. Adjust the balance of vinegar and oil according to your preference.

3. Emulsify: Whisk vigorously until the ingredients are well combined and the dressing has emulsified.

4. Serve or Store: Use immediately, or store in an airtight container in the refrigerator. The dressing will keep well for up to a week. Shake well before using if separated.

PREP TIME

5 MINUTES

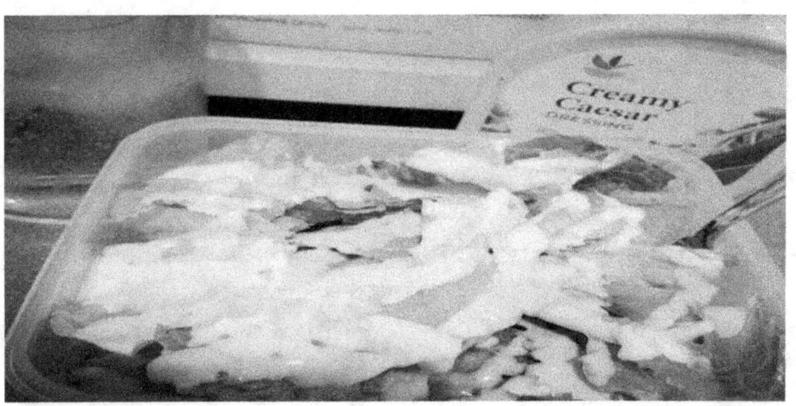

INGREDIENTS:

1/2 cup Greek yogurt (or mayonnaise for a more traditional version)

1/4 cup grated Parmesan cheese

1 clove garlic, minced

2 anchovy fillets, minced (or 1 teaspoon anchovy paste)

2 tablespoons lemon juice

1 teaspoon Dijon mustard

1 teaspoon Worcestershire sauce

1/4 cup olive oil

Salt and pepper, to taste

METHODS:

1. Combine Ingredients: In a bowl, whisk together Greek yogurt, Parmesan cheese, minced garlic, minced anchovies, lemon juice, Dijon mustard, and Worcestershire sauce.

2. Add Oil: Slowly drizzle in the olive oil while continuously whisking until the dressing is well-emulsified and creamy.

3. Season: Add salt and pepper to taste. Adjust the seasoning and acidity as needed.

4. Serve or Store: The dressing can be used immediately or stored in an airtight container in the refrigerator for up to a week.

PREP TIME

10 MINUTES

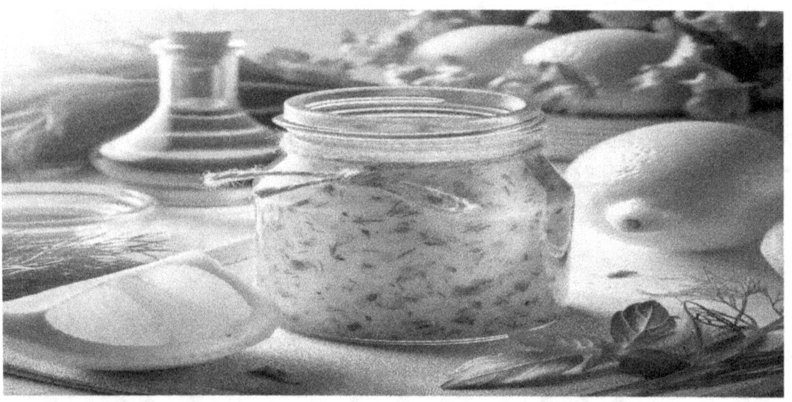

INGREDIENTS:

1/4 cup fresh lemon juice

1/2 cup olive oil

1 clove garlic, minced

1 tablespoon fresh parsley, finely chopped

1 tablespoon fresh dill, finely chopped

1 teaspoon honey or agave syrup (optional, for sweetness)

Salt and pepper, to taste

METHODS:

1. Combine Ingredients: In a small bowl or jar, whisk together lemon juice, olive oil, minced garlic, parsley, dill, and honey or agave syrup if using.

2. Season: Add salt and pepper to taste. Adjust the acidity or sweetness according to your preference.

3. Emulsify: Whisk or shake vigorously until the ingredients are well combined and the dressing is slightly emulsified.

4. Serve or Store: Use the dressing immediately, or store it in the refrigerator in an airtight container for up to a week. Shake well before using if it separates.

PREP TIME

5 MINUTES

28. Honey Mustard Glaze

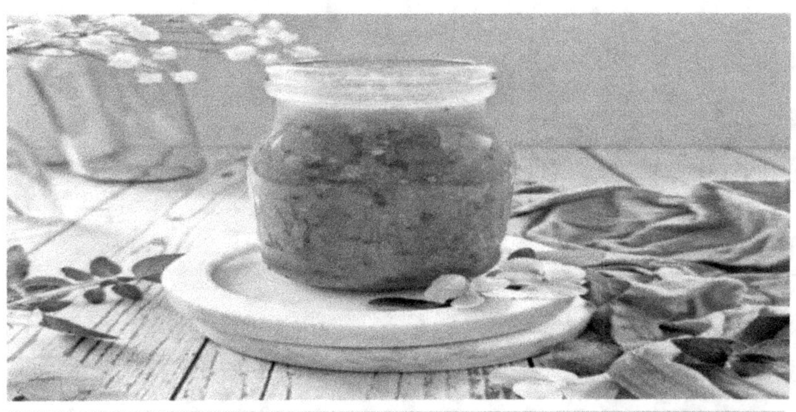

INGREDIENTS:

1/4 cup honey

1/4 cup Dijon mustard

1 tablespoon apple cider vinegar

1 teaspoon soy sauce

1 clove garlic, minced

Salt and pepper, to taste

PREP TIME

5 MINUTES

METHODS:

1. Combine Ingredients: In a small bowl, whisk together honey, Dijon mustard, apple cider vinegar, soy sauce, and minced garlic.

2. Season: Add salt and pepper to taste. Adjust the balance of honey and mustard according to your preference.

3. Use or Store: The glaze can be used immediately, or it can be stored in an airtight container in the refrigerator for up to two weeks.

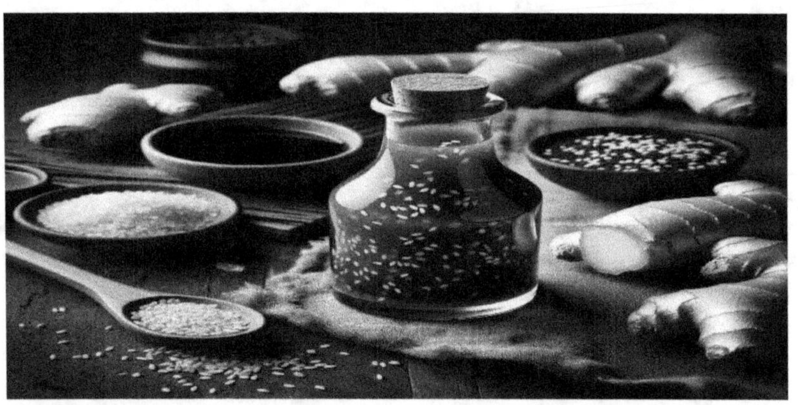

INGREDIENTS:

1/4 cup soy sauce

2 tablespoons sesame oil

2 tablespoons rice vinegar

1 tablespoon honey or agave syrup

1 tablespoon fresh ginger, grated

1 clove garlic, minced

1 teaspoon toasted sesame seeds

Optional: 1-2 teaspoons chili flakes or chili oil for heat

METHODS:

1. Combine Ingredients: In a small bowl or jar, whisk together soy sauce, sesame oil, rice vinegar, honey or agave syrup, grated ginger, and minced garlic.

2. Add Sesame Seeds: Stir in the toasted sesame seeds and chili flakes or chili oil if using.

3. Emulsify: Shake or whisk vigorously until all the ingredients are well combined and the dressing is slightly emulsified

4. Serve or Store: Use immediately or store in the refrigerator in an airtight container for up to a week. Shake well before use if it separates.

COOKING & PREP TIME

10 MINUTES

CHAPTER 8

Artisan Breads

The Come Hungry Cookbook delves into the realm of Artisan Breads in its eighth chapter. These bread recipes are more than just a means of subsistence; they are works of art, a sensory experience, and a celebration of the beauty that can be achieved from basic ingredients when prepared with skill and patience.

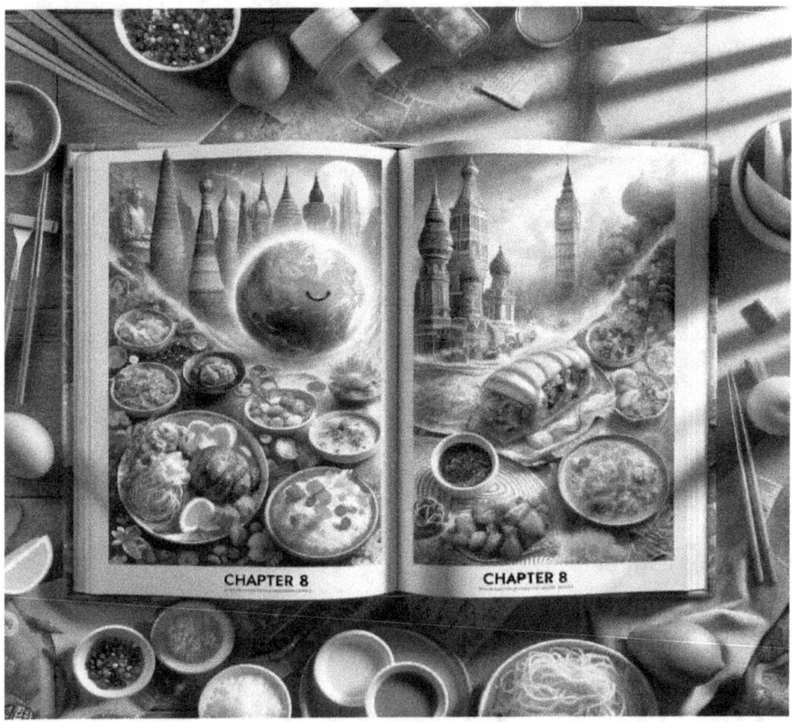

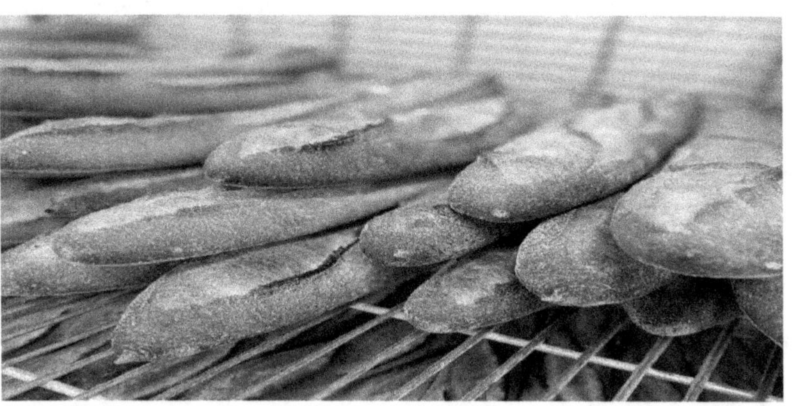

INGREDIENTS:

4 cups all-purpose flour

1 teaspoon salt

1 teaspoon instant yeast

1 1/3 cups warm water

COOKING & PREP TIME

145 MINUTES

METHODS:

1. Mix Dough: In a large bowl, mix the flour, salt, and yeast. Gradually add warm water and stir until a shaggy dough forms.

2. Knead: Turn the dough onto a lightly floured surface and knead for about 10 minutes, until smooth and elastic.

3. First Rise: Place the dough in a lightly oiled bowl, cover it with a clean towel, and let it rise in a warm place for about 1 hour, or until doubled in size.

4. Shape Baguettes: Punch down the dough and divide It into two equal parts. Roll each piece into a long, thin shape, approximately 14 inches long.

5. Second Rise: Place the shaped baguettes on a baking sheet lined with parchment paper. Cover and let them rise for about 30 minutes.

6. Preheat Oven: Preheat your oven to 475°F (245°C). If available, place a baking stone in the oven to heat.

7. Score and Bake: Just before baking, make diagonal slashes along the top of each baguette. Spray the oven with water to create steam and place the baguettes in the oven. Bake for 25 minutes or until golden brown.

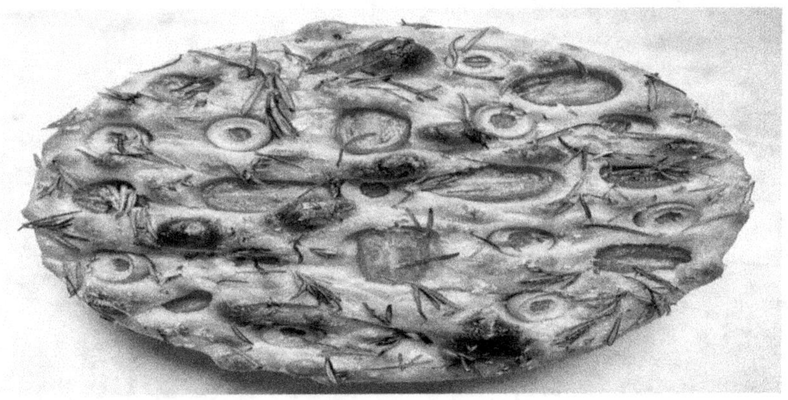

INGREDIENTS:

2 1/2 cups all-purpose flour

1 teaspoon salt

1 teaspoon instant yeast

1 cup warm water

1/4 cup olive oil, plus more for drizzling

2 tablespoons fresh rosemary, chopped

Coarse sea salt, for sprinkling

COOKING & PREP TIME

120 MINUTES

METHODS:

1. Prepare Dough: In a large bowl, mix the flour, salt, and yeast. Add warm water and 1/4 cup olive oil. Stir until a sticky dough forms.

2. First Rise: Cover the bowl with a damp cloth and let the dough rise in a warm place for about 1 hour, or until doubled in size.

3. Shape Dough: Gently press the dough into a greased 9x13-inch baking pan, spreading it evenly. Cover and let it rise for another 20 minutes.

4. Preheat Oven: Preheat your oven to 400°F (200°C).

5. Add Toppings: Use your fingers to dimple the top of the dough. Drizzle with olive oil and sprinkle with chopped rosemary and coarse sea salt.

6. Bake: Bake in the preheated oven for 20-25 minutes or until golden brown.

7. Cool and Serve: Serve warm

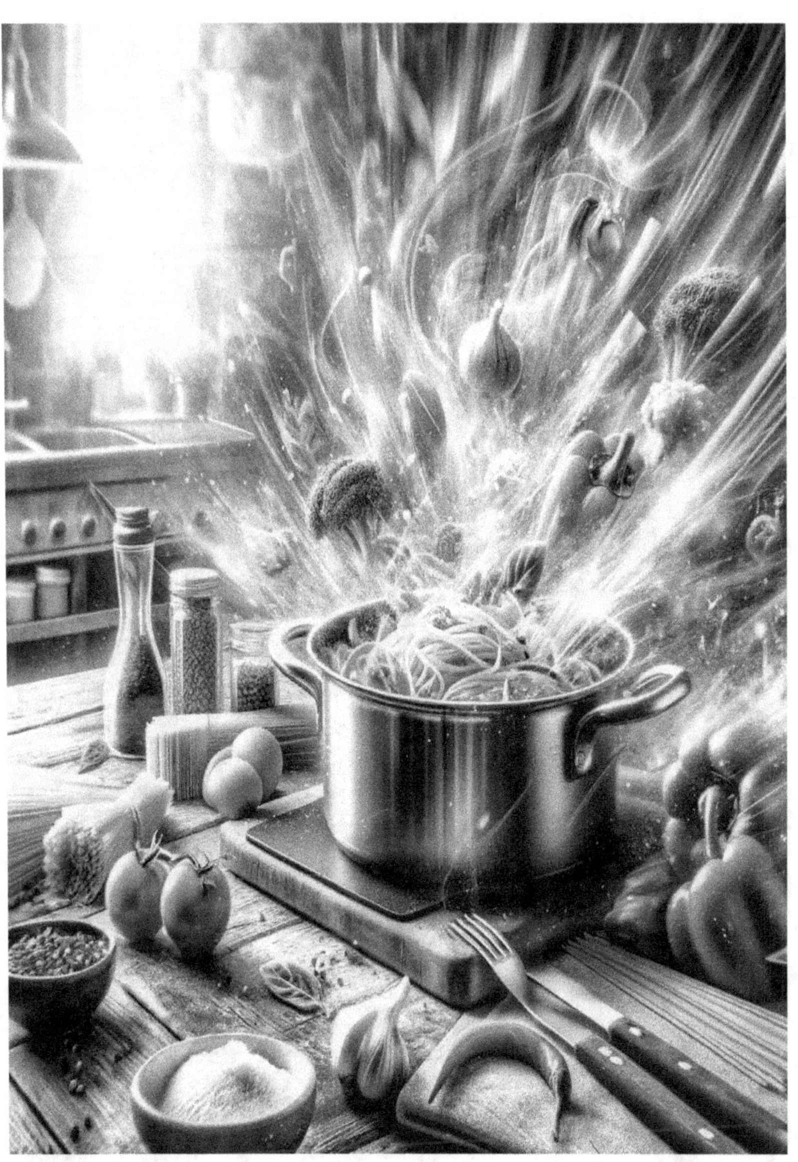

CHAPTER 9

Kitchen Essentials

In the "Come Hungry Cookbook," we explore the realm of Kitchen Essentials in chapter nine. These are the ingredients and methods that any home cook should have on hand because they are the fundamentals of culinary creativity. This chapter gives you the tools to use basic ingredients to enrich your cuisine, from handmade broths to crucial sauces.

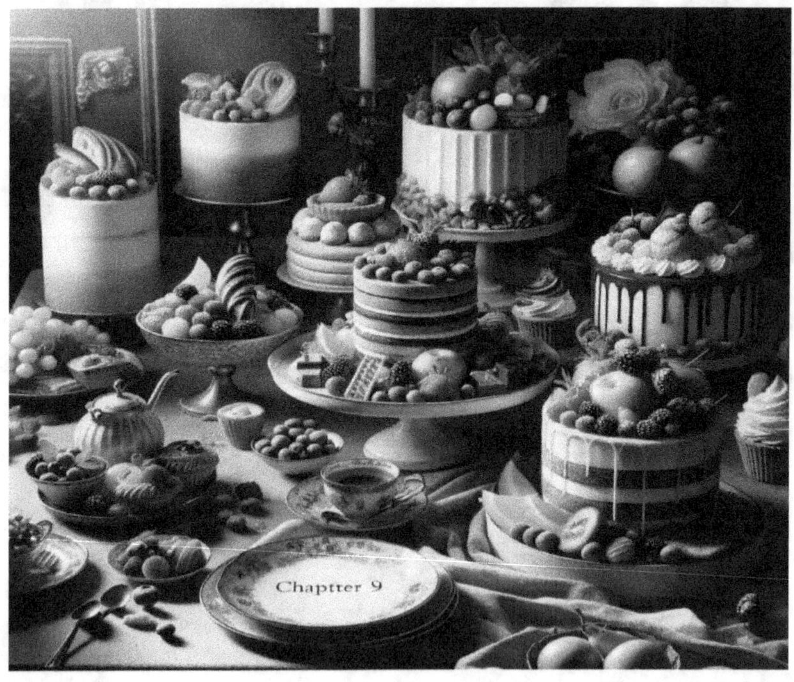

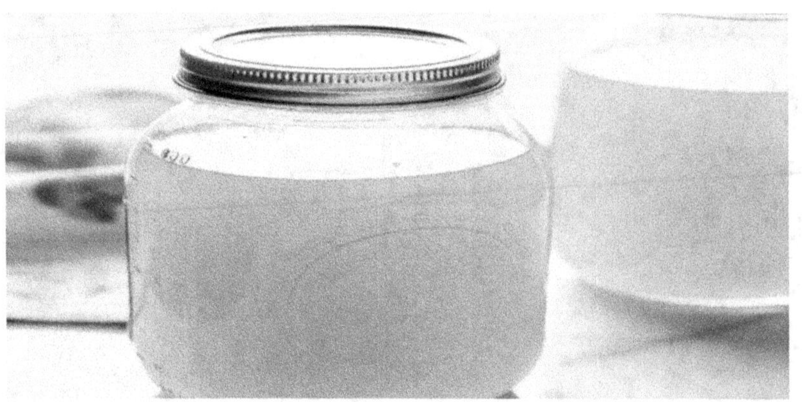

INGREDIENTS:

1 whole chicken carcass (leftover from a roasted or rotisserie chicken)

2 carrots, chopped

2 celery stalks, chopped

1 large onion, quartered

4 cloves garlic, smashed

2 bay leaves

A few sprigs of fresh thyme or parsley

1 teaspoon whole peppercorns

Salt, to taste

Water

COOKING & PREP TIME

255 MINUTES

METHODS:

1. Prepare Ingredients: Place the chicken carcass in a large stockpot. Add carrots, celery, onion, garlic, bay leaves, thyme or parsley, and peppercorns.

2. Add Water: Fill the pot with enough water to cover the ingredients by a couple of inches.

3. Simmer: Bring the mixture to a boil over high heat. Once boiling, reduce the heat to low and let it simmer, partially covered, for 3-4 hours. Skim off any foam or fat that rises to the surface.

4. Strain: After simmering, strain the broth through a fine-mesh sieve into a large container, discarding the solids.

5. Season: Add salt to taste and let the broth cool.

6. Store the broth in the fridge for 5 days

33. Basic Tomato Sauce

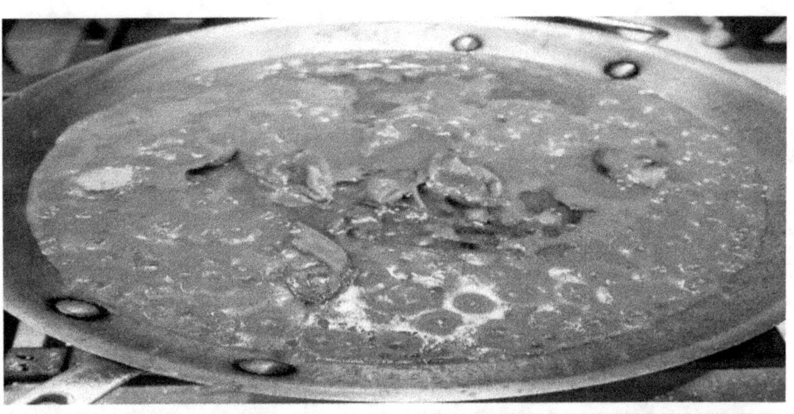

INGREDIENTS:	METHODS:

2 tablespoons olive oil

1 large onion, finely chopped

4 cloves garlic, minced

1 can (28 ounces) crushed tomatoes

1 teaspoon sugar (optional, to balance acidity)

1 teaspoon dried basil

1 teaspoon dried oregano

Salt and pepper, to taste

Fresh basil or parsley for garnish (optional)

COOKING & PREP TIME

40 MINUTES

1. Sauté Aromatics: In a large saucepan, heat the olive oil over medium heat. Add the chopped onion and sauté until translucent. Add the minced garlic and cook for another minute.

2. Add Tomatoes: Pour in the crushed tomatoes. Stir in sugar (if using), dried basil, and oregano.

3. Simmer: Bring the sauce to a simmer. Reduce the heat to low and let it simmer, uncovered, for about 25-30 minutes. Stir occasionally.

4. Season: Season the sauce with salt and pepper to taste.

5. Garnish & Serve: If using, garnish with fresh basil or parsley. Use immediately, or allow it to cool and store in the fridge or freezer for later use.

34. Classic Bechamel Sauce

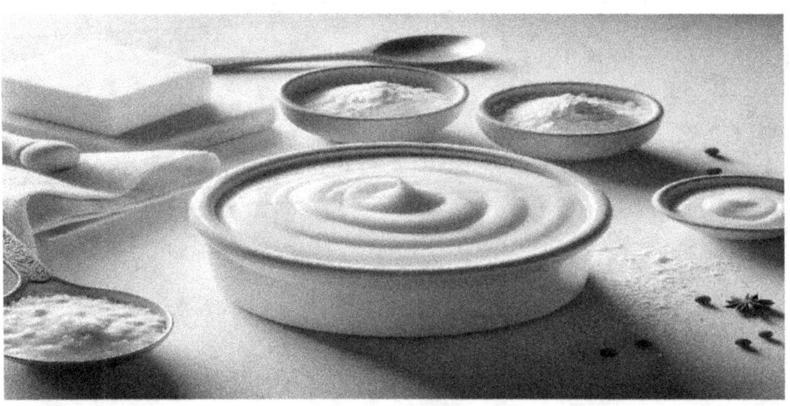

INGREDIENTS:

2 tablespoons unsalted butter

2 tablespoons all-purpose flour

2 cups whole milk, warmed

Salt and white pepper, to taste

Nutmeg, a pinch (optional)

METHODS:

1. Make Roux: In a medium saucepan, melt the butter over medium heat. Add the flour and whisk continuously for about 2 minutes to form a roux. Be careful not to let it brown.

2. Add Milk: Gradually add the warm milk, whisking constantly to prevent lumps. Continue to cook and whisk until the sauce thickens and starts to simmer.

3. Season: Lower the heat and simmer for a few more minutes. Season with salt, white pepper, and a pinch of nutmeg if desired.

4. Strain (Optional): For an ultra-smooth sauce, strain it through a fine-mesh sieve.

5. Use the béchamel sauce immediately. It can be refrigerated for up to 3 days.

COOKING & PREP TIME

15 MINUTES

35. Homemade Pesto

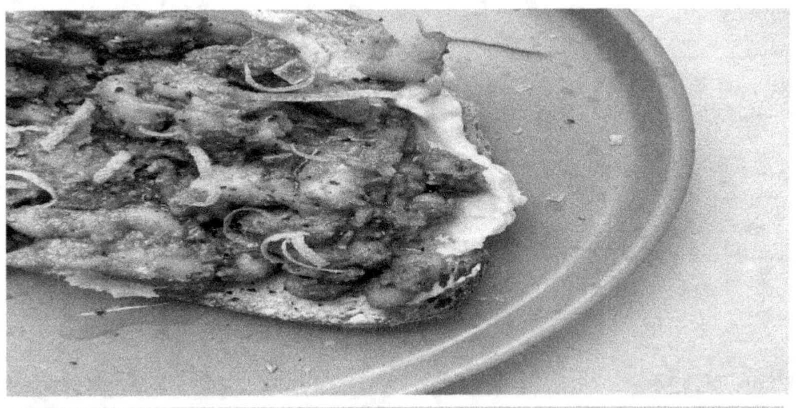

INGREDIENTS:

2 cups fresh basil leaves, packed

1/3 cup pine nuts (can substitute with walnuts or almonds)

3 cloves garlic

1/2 cup extra-virgin olive oil

1/2 cup grated Parmesan cheese

Salt and pepper, to taste

Lemon juice (optional, for added brightness)

METHODS:

1. Blend Ingredients: In a food processor or blender, combine the basil leaves, pine nuts, and garlic. Pulse until coarsely chopped.

2. Add Oil: With the processor running, slowly pour in the olive oil and process until the mixture is smooth.

3. Mix in Cheese: Transfer the mixture to a bowl. Stir in the grated Parmesan cheese. Add salt, pepper, and lemon juice (if using) to taste.

4. Serve or Store: Use the pesto immediately, or store it in an airtight container in the refrigerator with a layer of olive oil on top to preserve freshness. It can be stored for up to a week.

COOKING & PREP TIME

10 MINUTES

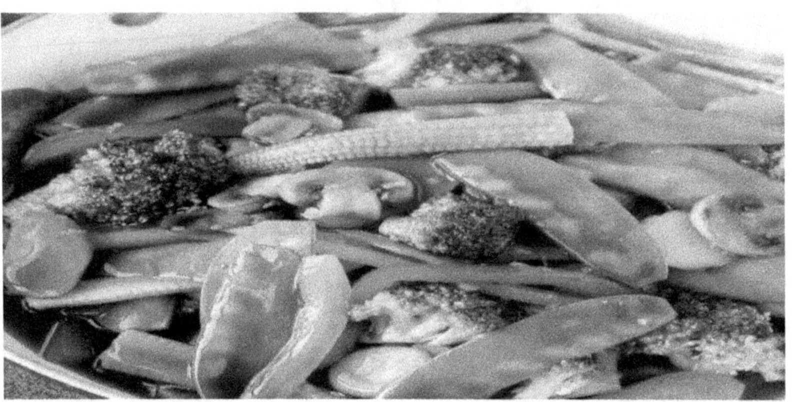

INGREDIENTS:

1 onion, quartered (no need to peel)

2 carrots, chopped

2 celery stalks, chopped

4 cloves garlic, smashed (no need to peel)

1-cup vegetable scraps (like mushroom stems, bell pepper cores, etc.)

2 bay leaves

A few sprigs of fresh parsley or thyme

1-teaspoon whole peppercorns

8 cups water

Salt, to taste (optional)

COOKING & PREP TIME

75 MINUTES

METHODS:

1. Prepare Ingredients: In a large stockpot, combine onion, carrots, celery, garlic, vegetable scraps, bay leaves, parsley or thyme, and peppercorns.

2. Add Water: Pour in water. The water should cover the vegetables by a couple of inches.

3. Simmer: Bring the mixture to a boil over high heat. Once boiling, reduce the heat to low and let it simmer, uncovered, for about 1 hour.

4. Strain: After simmering, strain the stock through a fine-mesh sieve into a large container, discarding the solids.

5. Add salt to taste, if desired, and let the stock cool. Store the stock in the fridge for a week

CHAPTER 10

DIY Kitchen Staples

In this last chapter of the "Come Hungry Cookbook," we go into the realm of do-it-yourself kitchen staples. These are the home-cooked components that take your cooking to the next level and let you make dishes with distinctive flavors and individual touches. This chapter gives you the tools to elevate your culinary creations, from spice blends to condiments.

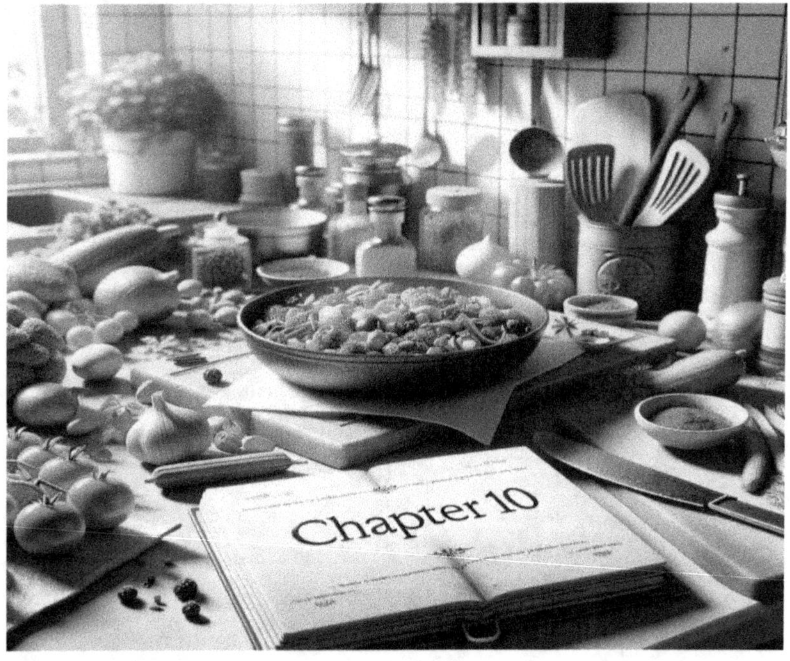

37. Homemade Mayonnaise

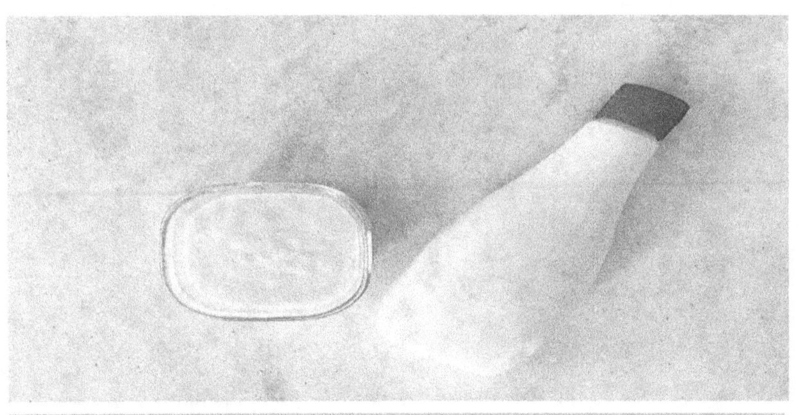

INGREDIENTS:

1 large egg yolk, room temperature

1 tablespoon Dijon mustard

1 tablespoon red or white wine vinegar or lemon juice

1 cup olive oil or avocado oil

Salt, to taste

Optional: A pinch of sugar or honey, garlic, or herbs for flavor

METHODS:

1. Blend Yolk & Seasonings: In a bowl, whisk together the egg yolk, mustard, and vinegar or lemon juice until well blended.

2. Add Oil Slowly: Slowly drizzle in the oil while continuously whisking. The mixture should start to thicken as you add more oil.

3. Season: Once all the oil has been incorporated and the mayonnaise is thick, season with salt and add any optional flavorings. Adjust acidity if needed by adding a bit more vinegar or lemon juice.

4. Storage: Store the mayonnaise in a sealed container in the refrigerator. Use within 3-5 days.

COOKING & PREP TIME

20 MINUTES

38. Zesty Taco Seasoning

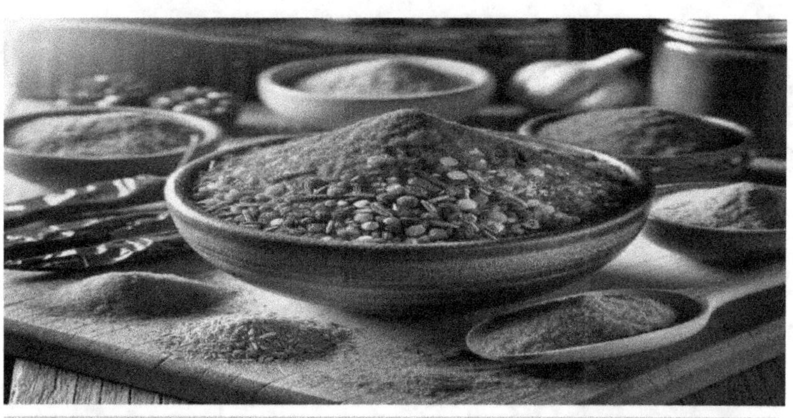

INGREDIENTS:

2 tablespoons chili powder

1 tablespoon ground cumin

2 teaspoons paprika (smoked or regular)

1 teaspoon garlic powder

1 teaspoon onion powder

1 teaspoon dried oregano

1 teaspoon crushed red pepper flakes (adjust to taste)

1 teaspoon black pepper

1-2 teaspoons salt (adjust to taste)

METHODS:

1. Combine Spices: In a small bowl, mix the chili powder, cumin, paprika, garlic powder, onion powder, oregano, red pepper flakes, black pepper, and salt until well combined.

2. Store: Transfer the seasoning mix to an airtight container or spice jar. Store in a cool, dry place.

COOKING & PREP TIME

10 MINUTES

39. Fresh Basil Pesto

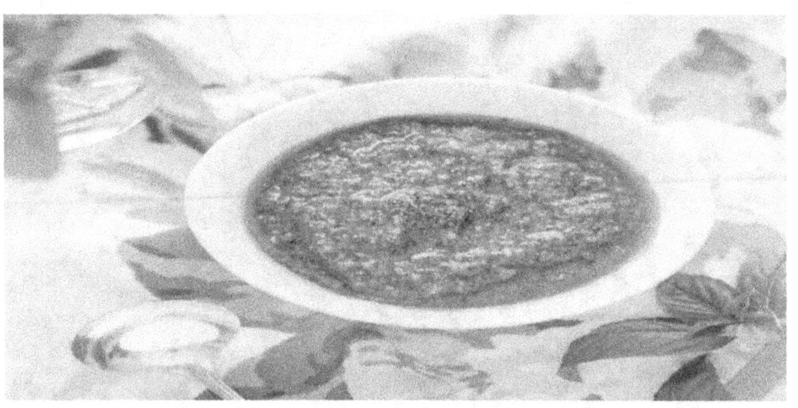

INGREDIENTS:

2 cups fresh basil leaves, packed

1/2 cup Parmesan cheese, freshly grated

1/2 cup extra virgin olive oil

1/3 cup pine nuts (can substitute walnuts or almonds)

3 garlic cloves, minced

Salt and pepper, to taste

Optional: a squeeze of lemon juice

COOKING & PREP TIME

20 MINUTES

METHODS:

1. Blend Basil and Nuts: In a food processor, blend basil leaves and pine nuts until coarsely chopped.

2. Add Garlic and Cheese: Add minced garlic and Parmesan cheese to the mixture and blend again.

3. Emulsify with Oil: While the food processor is running, slowly add the olive oil in a steady stream until the pesto is emulsified and reaches your desired consistency.

4. Season: Season with salt and pepper to taste. Add a squeeze of lemon juice if desired for extra freshness.

5. Store or Serve: Use immediately, or store in the refrigerator for up to a week. For longer storage, pesto can be frozen in an airtight container.

40. Roasted Red Pepper Sauce

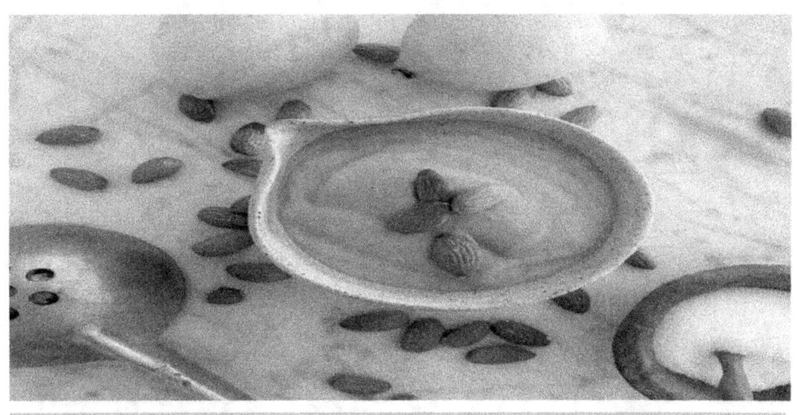

INGREDIENTS:

3 large red bell peppers

2 tablespoons olive oil

1 small onion, chopped

3 cloves garlic, minced

1/2 cup vegetable broth or water

1 teaspoon smoked paprika

1/2 teaspoon red pepper flakes (optional)

Salt and black pepper to taste

2 tablespoons fresh basil or parsley, chopped

COOKING & PREP TIME

45 MINUTES

METHODS:

1. Roast Peppers: Preheat oven to 450°F (230°C). Roast whole red peppers on a baking sheet for 25-30 minutes until charred. Cool in a covered bowl for 10-15 minutes, then peel and deseed.

2. Prepare Sauce: In a saucepan, heat olive oil over medium heat. Sauté onion and garlic for 5 minutes. Add roasted peppers, smoked paprika, red pepper flakes (optional), and vegetable broth. Season with salt and pepper. Simmer for 10 minutes.

3. Blend: Puree the sauce until smooth using a blender or immersion blender. Return to pan and reheat, adjusting seasoning as needed.

4. Stir in chopped basil or parsley. Serve over pasta or grilled meats

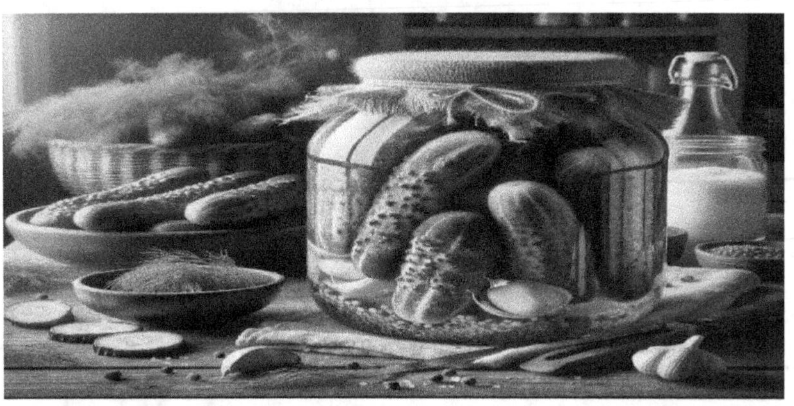

INGREDIENTS:

1-pound fresh cucumbers (preferably Kirby or Persian)

1 1/2 cups white vinegar

1 1/2 cups water

2 tablespoons pickling salt or kosher salt

4 garlic cloves, peeled and crushed

2 teaspoons dill seeds or 4 dill sprigs

1-teaspoon mustard seeds (optional)

1/2 teaspoon red pepper flakes

COOKING & PREP TIME

15 MINUTES

METHODS:

1. Sterilize jars and lids in boiling water for 10 minutes or in a dishwasher.

2. Wash and slice cucumbers as desired.

3. Make brine by boiling vinegar, water, and salt (add sugar for sweetness if desired).

4. Place dill, garlic, mustard seeds, and red pepper flakes in jars.

5. Pack cucumbers tightly into jars.

6. Pour hot brine over cucumbers, leaving 1/2 inch headspace.

7. Seal jars and let cool to room temperature.

8. Refrigerate for at least 24 hours before consuming.

9. Enjoy your pickles as a crunchy addition to meals.

CONCLUSION

Now that we've reached the conclusion of Come Hungry Cookbook: let's take a moment to appreciate this amazing culinary journey that we've shared. The goal of creating this cookbook was to use simple, approachable dishes to introduce you to the diversity of world food. Every meal has been an exploration of different cultures and flavors, from the tart Homemade Pickles to the spicy Roasted Red Pepper Sauce.

We traversed continents, tasted the spices of Asia, felt the warmth of the Mediterranean sun in our dishes, and embraced the hearty comfort of American classics. These 41 recipes were chosen not just for their delightful flavors but also for their simplicity and the joy they bring to the cooking process. Whether you are a seasoned chef or a novice in the kitchen, these dishes were designed to be accessible, inviting you to experiment with new ingredients and techniques without intimidation.

The underlying message of this cookbook is one of culinary exploration and embracing diversity. Food is a universal language, speaking directly to our hearts and souls. It has the power to bring people together, open our minds, and enrich our lives with experiences and flavors previously unimagined. Each recipe in this book is a gateway to a new culture, a new taste, and a new perspective.

As you continue your culinary journey, remember that cooking is an art form marked by personal expression. Don't be afraid to adapt these recipes to your taste, to experiment with substitutions, or to add a personal twist. The kitchen is your canvas, and you are the artist. Let your palate guide you, your curiosity drives you, and your creativity inspires you.

In the spirit of this book, I encourage you not only to cook but also to share. Share your food, share your new-found knowledge, and share the joy that comes from a meal lovingly prepared. Invite friends over for a homemade dinner, teach a child one of these simple recipes, or bring a dish to a community event. In sharing, we strengthen our connections, broaden our horizons, and enrich our communities.

Come Hungry Cookbook was designed to inspire, motivate, and bring a slice of the world into your daily life. Keep exploring, keep tasting, and keep sharing.

Thank You Note

Dear Culinary Adventurers,

As we close the final pages of Come Hungry Cookbook: I want to extend a heartfelt thank you for joining me on this flavorful journey. Your enthusiasm for exploring and embracing the diverse tastes of the world is what makes this cookbook truly special.

Your support is not just about trying recipes; it is about sharing a love for food and culture. Each dish you have prepared is a testament to your adventurous spirit and willingness to bring new tastes into your home. Whether you are cooking for yourself, your family, or your friends, you are creating more than just meals—you are crafting experiences, memories, and connections.

Thank you for allowing this cookbook to be a part of your culinary exploration. Your passion for cooking and learning is what inspires authors like me to keep creating and sharing. I am incredibly grateful for your support and am excited to see where your culinary adventures take you next.

Happy Cooking and Bon Appétit!
Warm regards,
Benedict Robinson
Author of Come Hungry Cookbook

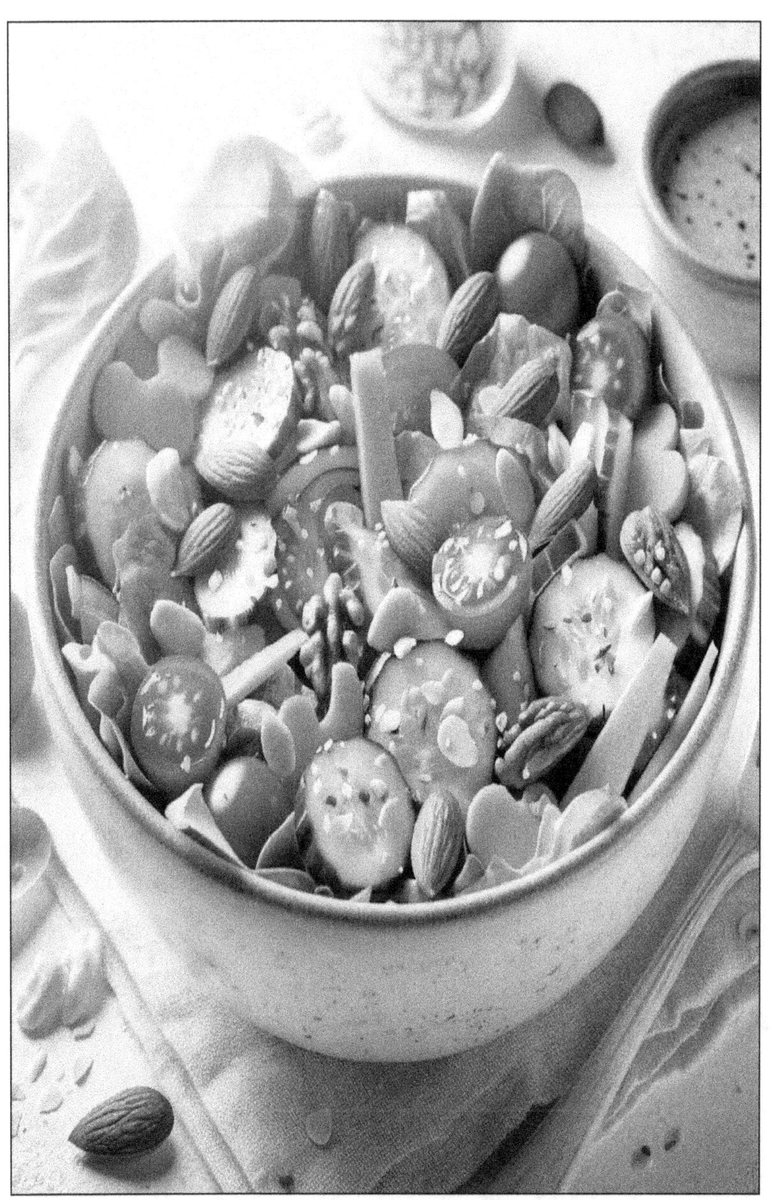

www.ingramcontent.com/pod-product-compliance
Lightning Source LLC
Chambersburg PA
CBHW050853260726
48660CB00006B/2612